CONTINUING NURSING EDUCATION

CONTINUING NURSING EDUCATION

Signe Skott Cooper, R.N., M.Ed.
Professor of Nursing
University of Wisconsin-Extension
University of Wisconsin, Madison, Wisconsin

May Shiga Hornback, R.N., Ph.D.
Professor of Nursing and
Chairman, Department of Nursing
University of Wisconsin-Extension
Madison, Wisconsin

McGraw-Hill Book Company

A Blakiston Publication

New York   St. Louis   San Francisco   Düsseldorf   Johannesburg
Kuala Lumpur   London   Mexico   Montreal   New Delhi   Panama
Rio de Janeiro   Singapore   Sydney   Toronto

Continuing Nursing Education

2 3 4 5 6 7 8 9 0 K P K P 7 9 8 7 6 5 4 3

Library of Congress Cataloging in Publication Data

Cooper, Signe Skott, 1921-
    Continuing nursing education.

    "A Blakiston publication."
    1. Nurses and nursing—Study and teaching—
United States. I. Hornback, May Shiga, 1924-
II. Title. [DNLM: 1. Education, Nursing,
Continuing. WY 18 C778c 1973]
RT81.U6C67   610.73'07'1   72-5089
ISBN 0-07-012940-1

This book was set in Theme by Creative Book Services,
division of McGregor & Werner, Incorporated. The editor
was Cathy Dilworth; the designer was Creative Book Services
and the production supervisor was Sally Ellyson.
The printer and binder was Kingsport Press, Inc.

Contents

Preface

The rapid pace of an ever-changing society and the continual alterations in practice resulting from modern technology present a challenge to the professional nurse. The challenge is even greater to nurse educators as they assist practicing nurses in their efforts to keep abreast of current developments in the nursing profession.

This book is designed primarily for nurse faculty members responsible for continuing education in institutions of higher learning. The authors believe that those institutions have an obligation to provide ongoing education to practicing nurses, and the book has been written to assist faculty members in carrying out this educational responsibility.

The authors recognize that hospitals and other health agencies have a responsibility for providing certain types of education to their employees and that professional and voluntary health agencies also carry responsibilities that may be designated as continuing education. Nurses employed in an educational capacity by these organizations will find much of the content of the book useful to them.

Both authors support the concept of self-directed learning and believe that faculty members in continuing education programs must first of all be continuing learners themselves. To help the faculty learner in his search for new knowledge and information extensive reference lists have been provided at the end of each chapter. We are aware that the nurse educator must also have a substantial nursing knowledge base, and we assume that readers are familiar with the great variety of clinical nursing learning resources now available.

The authors have had considerable experience in continuing education. The senior author was responsible for a statewide program of continuing education at the University of Wisconsin from 1955 until 1971. The co-author has been a member of the University of Wisconsin-Extension nursing faculty since 1965, and now directs the program. She has been primarily responsible for the use of new educational media in that program. This book is based on our experiences, and we are sharing what we are learning as pioneers in a field that is now rapidly expanding.

We acknowledge the assistance given by many persons, in particular the Wisconsin nurses who have consistently supported the program of the University of Wisconsin-Extension from its infancy, and who provided suggestions, encouragement, stimulation, and direction in the development of the program. Each faculty member of the Department of Nursing, University of Wisconsin-Extension, has contributed, directly and indirectly, to the content of this book. Two faculty members made special contributions: Shirley Adams, nursing specialist, gave many specific suggestions for Chapter 12, and Janet Nusinoff, assistant professor emeritus, read the entire manuscript. Nancy Nelson, administrative secretary in the department, typed the entire manuscript.

Burton W. Kreitlow, Professor of Educational Policy Studies and Agriculture and Extension Education, University of Wisconsin-Madison, deserves very special recognition for writing Chapter 3. He generously consented to write the chapter on very short notice. To have Dr. Kreitlow's contribution in this book is a pleasure and a privilege. Ranked among the foremost adult educators in the nation, Dr. Kreitlow has continued to serve on the Adult Education Association Commission of the Professors of Adult Education since its inception in 1955. The commissioners are dedicated to the improvement of the total field of adult education and Dr. Kreitlow personifies that dedication.

An increasing recognition of the importance of lifelong learning for professional nursing service will create new demands for supportive services. We hope this book will be of value to those persons who assist nurses in their never-ending quest for knowledge.

Signe Skott Cooper

May Shiga Hornback

CONTINUING NURSING EDUCATION

1

Why continuing education?

Rapid technologic advances, resulting from and related to the so-called knowledge explosion, have had an impact on every field of endeavor in recent years. The impact has been so great that continuing education has become an accepted way of life for many people, including some nurses. However, to some extent nursing as a profession has lagged behind other groups in recognizing the need for lifelong learning by the practitioner.

Certain exceptional nurses have always been self-directed learners. But most practitioners have generally accepted the trite statement "Once a nurse, always a nurse" almost as a slogan, reflecting the belief that nurses felt their education finished when they completed the basic nursing program. Indeed, there is some evidence that this very idea was taught in schools of nursing, sometimes directly, but usually in a more subtle manner.

The belief in the completeness of the education provided by the training school, as it was titled in the early history of nursing education, was prevalent enough to have been identified by one early writer on adult education. Charles Judd, in an article in a 1928 issue of the *American Journal of Nursing*, wrote: "I venture to advocate that the nursing profession give up the doctrine that a nurse is forever competent because at one time somebody put on her the stamp of approval as a graduate of a more or less adequately equipped training school." He continued, "... I am willing to assert that some continuation training in service for nurses would promote the well-being of the nation."[1]

In the last statement, Judd touched on a major reason for continuing education in nursing: the improvement of professional practice. This is the primary objective of programs in continuing education for nurses. Broadly speaking, however, lifelong learning in nursing relates not only to professional practice but also to the development of the person as an individual and as a responsible citizen.

As a citizen, the nurse shares with others a need to keep informed about the current issues of the day and to work constructively toward the solution of the serious problems confronting our society.

This book is written for nurses who are responsible for planning and administration of continuing education programs in nursing, and for those who teach in such programs. Designed in general for nurses who are faculty members of institutions of higher learning, the content will also be useful for nurses who are in-service educators in hospitals and other agencies.

Because the field of continuing education is very broad, reading this book may be profitable for many nurses who may not identify themselves as adult educators, but who in fact teach adults. Those nurses working with professional nursing groups, such as executive staffs of nursing organizations, as well as the members who volunteer for a myriad of education-related activities may be engaged in adult education. Nurses employed by the volunteer health agencies, such as heart associations, cancer societies, and mental health associations, are also responsible for continuing education programs.

The authors believe that nurses working with adults, individually and in groups, require a good understanding of the learner and his learning needs. The effective adult educator also uses teaching methods appropriate for the mature student. The two aspects of teaching are interrelated and are considered in this book.

DEFINITIONS

Definitions of some words which will be used throughout the book will help the reader understand more clearly the concepts discussed in the text.

Continuing education as defined by the *Dictionary of Education*, is "any extension of opportunities for reading, study and training to young persons and adults following their completion of or withdrawal from full-time school and college programs." In this dictionary continuing education is further defined as "education for adults provided by special schools, centers, colleges or institutes that emphasize flexible rather than traditional or academic programs "[2]

There are several definitions of *adult education* in the *Dictionary of Education*: "(1) Formal and informal instruction and aids to study for mature persons; (2) All activities with educational purposes carried on by mature persons on a part-time basis; (3) Any voluntary, purposeful effort toward the self-development of adults, conducted by public and private agencies, such as adult schools, extension centers, settlements, churches, clubs, and Chautauqua associations, for informational, cultural, remedial, vocational, recreational, professional, and other purposes."

Continuing education and *adult education* are often used interchangeably. However, we shall use the term continuing education. Historically, adult education was used to describe courses such as basic reading or mathematics to academically disadvantaged adults. To some extent this limited interpretation still persists, although now this type of education is usually described as *adult basic education.*

Continuing education sometimes encompasses formal academic study such as that in which a registered nurse may engage following the completion of a diploma program in nursing. Such education, frequently leading to a college degree, is continuing for the individual but will not be included for discussion in this book. For our purposes, the definition of *continuing nursing education* which appears in the *Nursing Thesaurus* of the *International Nursing Index* is useful: "Educational activities primarily designed to keep registered nurses abreast of their particular field of interest and do not lead to any formal advanced standing in the profession."[3]

In-service education is usually defined as a planned instructional or training program provided by an employing agency in the employment setting and is designed to increase competence in a specific area. In-service education is one aspect of continuing education, but the terms are not interchangeable.

The term *program* needs clarification since it is used in a variety of ways. In this book, program is used to describe planned, organized efforts directed toward accomplishing major objectives. A program includes many segments, which are described as educational activities or courses. The terminology becomes confusing in common usage, since a particular course may be referred to as a program.

Using the broad definition, a continuing education program offered by a nursing department is usually comprised of a number of different segments. Technically, a one-day conference is not a program, but it may be considered one aspect of an overall program.

The terms *institute, workshop,* and *conference* are frequently used interchangeably to suggest some type of short-term educational activity, but there are some differentiating features.

Institute, the oldest of these terms, suggests a meeting for formal instruction. The *Dictionary of Education* defines an institute as "a meeting of adults to consider a general or specific subject in a series of lectures, conferences, study groups, or similar sessions, usually confined to several successive days or weeks; organized and promoted by universities, colleges, or other educational institutions."[4] The term is considered somewhat old-fashioned today, and other terms such as conference or workshop may be substituted, even though the definition more accurately describes the teaching activity.

A *workshop,* as the name implies, is used to describe a meeting in which the participants work and learn together. Open discussion and exchange of ideas characterize the workshop.

A *conference* also involves group participation, usually aimed toward solving a specific problem. The term is used rather generally, however, as a substitute for the older word, institute.

The word *seminar* is sometimes rather loosely used to describe a conference or workshop. Strictly speaking, a seminar is a group discussion following the presentation of a research project. In a seminar the proponent of the project must defend his findings, and the discussion provides an opportunity for the evaluation of the research.

THE NEED FOR CONTINUING EDUCATION IN NURSING

Rapid scientific and technological advances have greatly altered the practice of nursing. As with the practice of medicine, the gap between scientific knowledge and its application grows wider each year as a result of multiple

Figure 1-1 Technologic advances place increasing demands on nurses for keeping practice current. (*University Hospitals, Madison, Wisconsin*)

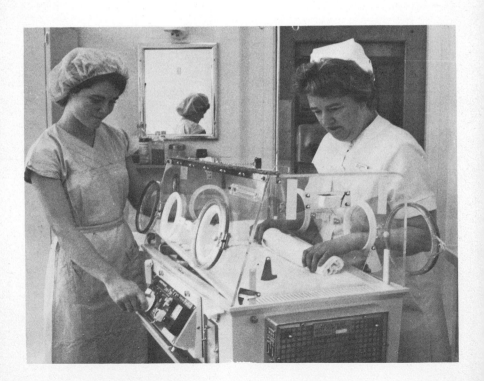

influences. The rapid advancement of research, the lack of easily accessible opportunities for continuing education, and the inefficient use of available means for the dissemination of knowledge are factors contributing to the gap.

A brief review of some of the medical progress of recent years provides an idea of the scope of the problem. The elimination of certain illnesses, particularly the communicable diseases, is within reach. New drugs have cured some illnesses, and altered the course of many others. Surgery is being performed successfully in areas that would not have been attempted ten to twenty years ago. Organ transplants have ceased to be a novelty. Complex and intricate machinery can extend lives. All these advances require more highly skilled nursing care in a great variety of settings.

The new techniques have created a multiplicity of associated problems, all of which demand nontraditional approaches. To cite one example, heart transplantation forced decisions relating to the determination of death. Ethical, moral, and legal issues are involved in making this decision and similar ones. Not only must medical personnel have broader knowledge and understanding to make rational and humane decisions, they must also be able to work with family members and nonprofessional advisory committees. New and different skills are required for effective decision making.

SIGNIFICANT SOCIAL TRENDS

Directly and indirectly, changes in nursing practice result from alterations in the society the profession serves. Changes in the delivery of health care will result from public demands for better care. It may be helpful to examine some of the present social trends that will influence nursing and health care.

Population Mobility

The migration of many people from one part of the country to another is a phenomenon observable since World War II. In hospitals and other health agencies mobility results in a high turnover of nursing personnel.

At one time the majority of staff nurses in many hospitals were graduates of that institution's school of nursing; they were familiar with all the details of the practice expected from them. Today the nurses come from many different institutions, often staying in one employment setting for only a short period of time. Hospitals have been forced to provide orientation and in-service education programs for employees with varying educational and experiential backgrounds.

Shifts in Age Composition

The proportion of the population age 65 and over continues to increase. For the nation as a whole about 10 percent of the population is in this age category.

The elderly are often plagued with various chronic illnesses and require nursing attention, both in and out of institutions. The number of nursing homes is increasing, but staffing them is often difficult. Furthermore, many nurses are ill-prepared to care for these patients, since basic educational programs have often been deficient in geriatric nursing content.

Increases associated with a general rise in the population are also evident in the group at the opposite end of the age scale: the very young. In 1965, 10 percent of the population was under the age of 5. Both age groups, the young and old, require much nursing care, and the need for better-prepared nurses to meet these demands is apparent.

Increasing Governmental Involvement in Health Care

More federal legislation relating to health has been passed by Congress during the last ten years than during our entire previous history. Such governmental involvement, both state and federal, will continue in the future.

Federal legislation has led to the development of many different public health programs; to the building of hospitals, nursing homes, and mental health centers; to hospital care for the nation's veterans; to substantial research on the crippling and killing diseases. Recent amendments to the Social Security Act have provided medical care to the elderly and to others unable to provide for themselves.

Standards set by the federal legislation have had an impact on the quality of care provided. Meeting the standards often requires some type of continuing education for practitioners.

Governmental involvement in health results in increasing demands for nursing care in many areas. Federal funds assist in the preparation of nurses to meet such demands and have been available for a number of years for the education of various categories of nursing personnel. Federally funded programs are discussed in more detail in later chapters.

The Changing Role of the Hospital

The traditional role of the hospital as a haven for the ill is being expanded to include a wide variety of preventive programs. The hospital of the future will function as a health center, reaching out into the community it serves.

The nurse in such a hospital will have a significant role, vastly different from the traditional one, and he will require a broader preparation for his responsibilities. The nurse of tomorrow will require a deeper knowledge of prevention and rehabilitation; a greater understanding of people and their problems; more ability in teaching patients; greater skill in working with many different groups of workers, including those who come from a variety of economic and cultural backgrounds. Additional preparation on and off the job will be required to help him fulfill this role adequately.

Mental Illness and Mental Health

Mental illness is the nation's number one health problem. It is predicted that one out of every ten persons in this country will spend some time in a mental hospital. Over half the hospital beds in this country are for the mentally ill. Yet less than 5 percent of the nation's nurses are employed in psychiatric institutions. [5]

Current developments in the care of the mentally ill emphasize the need for more and better-prepared psychiatric nurses. The inclusion of increasing numbers of psychiatric units in general hospitals and the establishment of more diagnostic and treatment centers pinpoint this need. The widespread increase in community health centers requires nurses with skills in individual and family counseling and therapy.

More attention directed to the promotion of positive mental health would alter the present depressing statistics. More knowledge and understanding is required by both health personnel and the lay public to effect change.

Maternal and Infant Mortality

It is sometimes said that the degree of civilization of any country can be measured by its maternal and infant death rates. The United States stands eleventh in a listing of the countries in the world in infant mortality—surely a disgrace in a country that prides itself on its medical knowledge and skill.

New knowledge and advances in technology have resulted in better means of caring for the prematurely born and high-risk infant. Nurses have a significant role here, both in preventive aspects and in caring for those at risk. The advancement of the science of genetics and the increasing concern and new methods for family planning suggest new teaching roles for nurses.

Changing Patterns in the Employment of Women

Since the vast majority of nurses are females, changing employment patterns among women are pertinent. More women are now employed than ever before in the history of this country, and among those employed, a higher proportion are married. At the same time, women are marrying at an earlier age.

The woman nurse graduating from a school of nursing today usually expects to combine marriage and a career, but large numbers leave the field, at least temporarily, after having had only a limited amount of nursing practice. Unless effective ways can be found to assist nurses who leave active practice to keep in touch professionally, it may be difficult to entice them back to practice. Effective continuing education can help influence an individual's decision.

The number of married nurses has increased steadily over the past 25 years, so that today 64 percent of employed nurses are married. [6] Today's nurse is torn by the many challenges facing her in the complex role as a member of a profession, as a key person in the family structure, and as a responsible citizen. She may be vitally interested in keeping professionally informed, but the effort required may be too taxing. Thus, new approaches to helping her learn in a setting near her home are indicated.

Part-time work is associated with the increase in employment among women. Driven by necessity, hospitals have been in the vanguard in providing these employment opportunities. Indeed, many hospitals would not be able to function without a cadre of part-time nurses, and in 1966 about one-third of employed nurses in the nation worked less than full-time.

Very often the nurse who works part-time has special learning needs. Her work schedule may preclude her from the hospital's regular in-service education program and other learning opportunities. Because of family and other commitments, she often tends to take less responsibility for her own professional development.

The Inactive Nurse. The nurse who has been inactive for any period of time has special learning needs. However, as with illness, perhaps a preventive program is indicated. She needs assistance to prevent becoming so outdated that she cannot return to practice.

Rapidly changing nursing practices have made obsolete the tacit assumption that a nurse could always return to practice. Furthermore, as a greater proportion of schools of nursing have become tax-supported, questions are being raised about educating those who never intend to practice. In spite of many efforts to recruit men into the field, nursing remains primarily a women's occupation, and it can be predicted that varying periods of professional inactivity will be the life-style for a high proportion of nurses in the future.

The nursing profession has not given adequate consideration to ways of assisting nurses to keep updated during periods of inactivity. As a result, inactive nurses themselves have done very little to keep current. Except for sporadic reading and occasional refresher courses, significant continuing education efforts of this group have been minimal.

The rapid technologic advances preclude the possibility of keeping up with all the current developments in the profession. No matter how short the period of inactivity, nor how intensive the learning efforts during this time, the returning nurse will require an extensive orientation to the employment setting. But the transition back into nursing is more easily accomplished if the nurse is aware of current developments, is familiar with learning resources, and has well-established study patterns.

The inactive nurse is considered in more detail in Chapter 10, but is identified here as a large segment of the population with special learning needs. A broad program of continuing education in nursing must provide means of assisting the nonpracticing nurse to retain skills and gain new knowledge.

TRENDS IN THE PROVISION OF HEALTH CARE

Changes in the provision of care place increasing demands upon the educational systems preparing the practitioner. These changes are reflected in innovative curricula, such as those preparing nurses for primary care. But curriculum adjustment occurs slowly, and formal educational programs are not synchronized with current developments in practice. Thus increasing emphasis on the continuing education of the practitioner is required to meet increasing demands for changes in the delivery of health care.

In recent years, a crisis in health care has been identified in this country. It has not been accurately established if, in fact, this is more of a crisis than has been in existence for some time, or if it is due to the increasing visibility of groups which have never had adequate health care. Such groups include members of minorities (especially the economically and socially deprived members of minority groups), those living in certain geographic sections (particularly in rural areas), and the poor.

The identification of health care as a crisis resulted from a number of factors: rising costs of health and medical care, maldistribution of health manpower, inaccessibility of comprehensive medical care, and an increasing awareness by an informed public of the gaps in the present system of health care.

As a result of the concern over the health care crisis, increasing amounts of time and attention have been directed toward exploring innovative systems of health care delivery. New techniques for improving the effectiveness and efficiency of health personnel are required if the health needs of citizens are to be met. Continuing education for the maintenance of professional competence is necessary for developing innovative approaches to health care.

The establishment of regional medical programs across the entire country was one attempt directed toward solving the health care crisis. Although it may be true that the regional medical programs have not yet lived up to their promise, significant benefits—tangible and intangible—came from this nationwide effort. In many instances, regional medical programs promoted the development of continuing education for nurses, doctors, and allied health workers living in areas with limited educational opportunities. Of special note is the benefit gained by the various health professionals meeting and working together.

Speculation about the future delivery of health care is risky, since it will be influenced by the demand of the citizens, the economy of the country, health legislation, and other factors, but it seems fairly certain that alterations in the system of health care in this country will be forthcoming. The adoption of a system of national health insurance is one possible approach; several different plans are being promoted by various interest groups.

Another possible development is the expansion of Health Maintenance Organizations (HMOs). This organization for health care permits a long overdue shift in emphasis from acute episodic care to the maintenance of health. Various organizations may follow different structural patterns, but each is based on a system of health care that provides for health maintenance and treatment services to an enrolled population. Members pay a fixed annual sum for the service. Although the HMO is not limited to group practice, this is the usual structural model.

However health care is provided in the future, the practitioner will require some type of continuing education to function effectively and efficiently. If health maintenance organizations are to live up to their names, the emphasis must be on health maintenance, health teaching, and prevention of illness of members. Here nurses can make a special and unique contribution, but only if they are prepared for a new and different role, and only if that role is clearly understood by all those involved, including the participating members of the organization. Continuing education is required by the staff and members alike.

The establishment of Area Health Education Centers, as recommended by the Carnegie Commission on Higher Education, will provide more easily accessible continuing education for many different health workers. Cooperative arrangements between these centers located in institutions of higher learning and university medical centers will provide a means of more rapid application of research findings to practice.

The Changing Nature of Nursing

Technological advances and related medical developments have had and will continue to have a profound influence on nursing. The day of the all-purpose nurse appears to be over. No longer can the new graduate be expected to function as a polished practitioner in any setting as soon as he leaves the school of nursing.

The basic education of the nurse does not provide adequate preparation for certain positions in the broad areas of community health. Increasingly, nursing curriculums are being designed to prepare graduates for practice outside the hospital, but many nurses are now being employed in areas for which they are inadequately prepared. Examples include the nurse employed in industry, in schools, in a home care or generalized public health agency. Furthermore, these agencies often have a very small staff, so in-service education is extremely limited. The situation demands some other type of continuing education.

All too often, positions in nursing are filled by those inadequately prepared for the demands of the job. Examples abound in every area of nursing practice: head nurses and supervisors, in-service educators, teachers in various educational programs. Often nurses filling these positions are searching for ways to upgrade their practice. Short courses and other continuing education activities can assist them in discharging their responsibilities more effectively.

Clinical Content. Another obvious deficit is in the area of clinical content. Nurses whose clinical responsibilities are rapidly changing require many different approaches, on the job and elsewhere, for meeting their learning needs. Educational opportunities in the clinical setting are not always recognized or used to good advantage.

Nurses may also leave one area of nursing practice for another. Entering an unfamiliar area of practice with insufficient preparation creates obvious learning needs. This may be particularly troublesome when the nurse enters an area, such as geriatric nursing, where clinical knowledge has not been advanced to the degree required for excellence in practice.

Technological advances demand highly specialized nursing knowledge and skill in areas such as the intensive care unit, the coronary care unit, the hemodialysis unit, or the emergency suite. Short term preparatory courses have emphasized the technical aspects of care, but additional education is required to assist the nurse to provide supportive care to patients with conditions having a deeply emotional overlay.

The Clinical Nurse Specialist. The advent of the nurse specialist was an important milestone for the profession, for it clarified the role of the professional nurse in the care of patients. It emphasized the importance of nursing care of patients, for the clinical nurse specialist is able to provide a highly sophisticated level of care.

The clinical specialist in nursing has a broad base of theoretical knowledge upon which to base nursing decisions and actions. This nurse has special skills in assessing and meeting nursing needs of patients. Responsibilities vary from one clinical setting to another, but include providing care to patients, and assisting others in evaluating and giving effective nursing care.

Unfortunately, qualified clinical nurse specialists are in short supply, and to date the unique contributions of these highly skilled practitioners are unknown in many parts of the country. Practice tends to be limited to large hospitals and medical centers but, as the role of this nurse is more fully understood and appreciated, opportunities will surely expand.

The nurse specialist who is adequately prepared educationally will seek ways to keep himself continually updated. The nurse who attempts to function in the specialist's role, but without formal preparation, will require many opportunities for continuing his education.

Auxiliary and Supportive Nursing Personnel. Much of the care provided to patients in hospitals and nursing homes is given by auxiliary personnel, and increasingly this is true in community health agencies. The quality of the care may suffer as the number of these workers reaches ever higher proportions, unless safeguards to patient care are established. Added responsibilities are placed on nurses for the supervision of these workers, but frequently nurses are not prepared for these supervisory functions. As a result, patient care is often less than satisfactory.

More effective utilization of all health workers is required for improved health care delivery. The general trend for the preservice training of nursing assistants and other workers in vocational schools has a positive effect on the nursing service received by patients. These training programs provide a more economical and more uniform system of education than that offered by most hospitals, but do not relieve the employing agency of its responsibility for orientation and ongoing in-service education for these workers.

New Roles for Health Workers

Although the number of nurses in relation to the population has been increasing since the turn of the century, the number of physicians has been decreasing. It is expected that the decline will continue, particularly in rural and economically disadvantaged areas. The impact on nursing has often been to thrust additional responsibilities on nurses whenever there is an inadequate medical staff. However, the shortage of nurses compounded the problem.

Increasing demands from all segments of society for more and better health care have resulted in exploration and experimentation with extended roles for nurses and the creation of new types of workers. At issue is the delivery of more effective care to larger numbers of people. The high cost of medical care is a related issue.

The Extended Role of the Nurse.   To some, any discussion of an extended role of the nurse is limited to the physician's assistant role. This may be a semantic distinction, and obviously the nurse functioning as a physician's assistant is in a role expanded beyond the traditional nursing one, but the concept of an extended role goes beyond merely that of an assistant to the physician.

The extended role of the nurse implies considerable independent functioning and decision making. It includes the performance of tasks that were once seen as solely the province of the physician. But it also requires considerable collaboration and team effort between the nurse and the physician.

The provision of primary care by the nurse is an extension of the traditional nursing role. This may be in such areas as the care of well infants and children, maintenance care of the chronically ill, limited psychotherapy and family counseling, health education and the promotion of positive health.

An extended role provides an opportunity for the nurse to use his own knowledge and skills in a more creative and productive way than is now possible. Some very exciting and challenging roles have emerged. The pediatric nurse practitioner, sometimes called the physician associate, is probably the most familiar example; training programs for this expanded role began at the University of Colorado in 1965.

The Physician's Assistant.   To many of its advocates, the use of the physician's assistant gave promise of a quick solution to an overwhelming problem. This new category of personnel was visualized as an answer to the problems resulting from an inadequate supply and maldistribution of physicians.

As the name implies, the physician's assistant works closely with and under the supervision of the physician. He is expected to do many of the repetitious and routine tasks of physicians, to permit the latter to do those tasks which only he can do. This idea is no different from the use of auxiliary nursing personnel to relieve the professional nurse of tasks which do not require professional skill and judgment.

Tasks assigned to the physician's assistant vary with his competence, knowledge, and training, and with the wishes of the particular physician with whom he works. As this role has evolved, three levels of workers are emerging:

1. Type A. This assistant will be trained to collect pertinent data, take patient histories, and perform diagnostic and therapeutic procedures. Preparation for this assistant is at the college level.

2. Type B. This assistant will possess exceptional skill in one clinical area, such as the renal dialysis unit. Training programs for these assistants are being established in technical colleges.

3. Type C. This assistant is trained to perform a variety of tasks under the direct supervision of the physician. He may have a minimum educational background, and is largely trained on the job.

Some nurses are employed as physician's assistants; they find satisfaction in this type of collaborative working relationship. Because of their previous education and experience, they can often be trained for this role in a minimum amount of time. As previously indicated, this is a different role, with considerably less independent function than the role of the physician associate. In either instance, additional and continuing education for the expected responsibilities are essential.

Technicians. Within the hospital, increasing types and numbers of technicians and related workers are being employed. These include such workers as the unit manager, the inhalation therapist, the surgical technician. The nurse must be able to work effectively with many different personnel.

The emergence of these technical workers can have a positive influence on total patient care. The inhalation therapist, for example, will have a greater depth of knowledge and more skill than many staff nurses. Conversely, additional workers result in more fragmented care, which requires greater skill by the nurse in the coordination of efforts for the good of the patient. This suggests further continuing education needs.

CURRENT DEVELOPMENTS IN CONTINUING EDUCATION

Since 1959, when the first short term courses were funded by the Division of Nursing, U.S. Public Health Service, increasing attention has been paid to continuing education by the Division. Details are given elsewhere in this book, but among the other examples that may be cited are the nationwide program for refresher courses for inactive nurses, the provision of support for special courses in coronary care, and the development of a multimedia system for teaching coronary care. Recent attention has been directed to supporting state and regional planning projects for continuing education in nursing.

In 1971 the Division of Nursing awarded the American Nurses' Association a grant to survey existing programs and resources for continuing education for registered nurses. The purpose of the survey was to assist the organization in planning to meet its responsibility in the area of continuing education for professional practice. This responsibility is seen as providing information about the availability of offerings as well as encouraging and facilitating the development of needed programs.

Continuing education for its members has always been one of the major purposes of the American Nurses' Association. However, a few recent significant developments may be noted. The ANA statement, "Avenues for Continued Learning," appeared in 1967. Three years later a new post of Coordinator of Continuing Education was established in the organization, and Audrey Spector was appointed to the position. In 1971 the ANA board of directors appointed a task force on continuing education; its purpose was to study the question of mandatory continuing education requirements for licensure. The next year a Council on Continuing Education was approved by the board; the Council will be under the Commission on Nursing Education within the Association.

State associations have also been concerned about continuing education, and in several instances, the question of continuing education requirements for membership has been seriously considered by these organizations. In at least three states, North Dakota, Arizona, and Utah, plans have been established for voluntary participation leading to recognition by members meeting the requirements. The continuing education requirements are delineated on a point system, and the nurse is expected to attain a specific number of points within a given period of time.

Such a system has merit, for it reflects the concern of the organization for the competence of its members to practice. Limitations of the system relate to difficulties in determining the quality of the educational offerings and their effect upon nursing practice. Since a precedent has been established in some states, others may soon follow.

Continuing Education Credit

The recent interest in continuing education credit raises some interesting philosophical questions. Are most nurses not adequately motivated to learn for the sake of learning or to improve their practice? Are outward symbols necessary to encourage nurses to learn? Is the establishment of continuing education requirements for relicensure the only way to prevent professional obsolescence in most practitioners? Should continuing education be required for merit increases on the job?

We live in a world where increasing emphasis is placed on status symbols, and academic credit is one of these symbols. In nursing, the significance of the college degree has often been so emphasized that the learning that occurs in the process of achieving the degree is seemingly devalued. This may explain why many nurses react negatively to noncredit courses: there is no outward recognition of achievement.

Certain types of continuing education activities, such as independent reading, cannot be measured, but this does not make the activity any less valuable to the learner. Even if a system of awarding some type of credit is established, these independent learning activities will remain an important aspect of self-development for the motivated learner.

The Continuing Education Unit. In 1968 a national conference was called to study the feasibility of a uniform unit of measurement for noncredit continuing education programs. The conference was sponsored by the U.S. Civil Service Commission, the U.S. Office of Education, the American Association of Collegiate Registrars and Admissions Officers, and the National University Extension Association. As a result of this conference, a national task force was created to consider the possibility of developing a uniform continuing education unit.

In an interim statement, the national task force defined the continuing education unit: Ten contact hours of participation in an organized continuing education experience under responsible sponsorship, capable direction, and qualified instruction.[7]

The continuing education unit will provide a mechanism for recording continuing education activities. The use of the unit is being tried in a pilot project in sixteen institutions, and following this study, recommendations will be made regarding more general use.

Participating institutions will be responsible for establishing and maintaining a permanent record of all continuing education units awarded. Records will include basic identification information, such as the name and social security number of the student, and information about the course: title, description, format, starting and ending date, and number of continuing education units awarded.

If continuing education becomes mandatory for membership in the professional association, for renewal of licensure, or for both, a system of record keeping becomes obligatory. The use of the continuing education unit would simplify records that an individual may wish to keep for his personal use.

Licensure Requirements

The relationship between continuing education and professional competence is obvious, but it is less clear how practitioners can be motivated to continue to learn. Increasingly, provisions for mandatory continuing education are being considered by licensing bodies.

The rationale underlying mandatory continuing education for relicensure is to protect the public by upgrading professional standards. This idea is not unique to nursing; for example, in many states teachers must present evidence of recent education to renew their teaching certificates. As a socially responsible and responsive profession, nursing must support ways of assuring competence of practitioners.

Those who advocate mandatory continuing education licensure requirements are convinced that this is the only way to assure upgrading nursing practice. They believe that requiring the nurse to participate in continuing education will result in learning and, therefore, in changed practice. An exposure to new ideas may be beneficial. In the past, establishing and maintaining educational standards in nursing has resulted in improved practice.

Others are less convinced of the value of mandatory requirements. Even though the nurse is forced to attend a required number of course hours, he may not learn in the process, since learning is tied so closely to motivation. Mandatory requirements do not account for individual differences in learning; many nurses learn a great deal in ways that are not measurable by the usual standards. These ways include reading, informal discussions with colleagues, independent investigation, trying out new approaches to care, case conferences, writing for publication, and so on.

In December 1971, legislation was passed in California requiring registered and licensed practical nurses to meet continuing education requirements for licensure renewal. This legislation takes effect in 1977. Although some states have similar requirements for the practice of pharmacy, dentistry, and other health professions, California is the first state requiring continuing education for the practice of nursing.

In debate on a resolution on continuing education at the House of Delegates session at the 1972 biennial convention of the American Nurses' Association, an amendment supporting mandatory continuing education was introduced but defeated. Nevertheless, with the precedent having been set in California, the question of mandatory continuing education is being investigated further in several states. At the present time the inclusion of mandatory continuing education requirements in state licensing laws would be premature in many parts of the country. Unless nurses have easy access to continuing education, such laws would be difficult to enforce and would place a hardship on many nurses.

It seems likely that nursing will follow the pattern of other health professions regarding licensure. Legislation pertaining to professional licensure is being intensively studied, nationally and in many states. Nurse educators will want to follow these developments closely, for action taken may substantially influence future educational practices.

If mandatory continuing education requirements become a reality, a means of accreditation of continuing education courses will be required. A means of determining relevancy of course content, and establishing standards and criteria for approved courses will need to be determined.

The issue of mandatory educational requirements will not be easily resolved since the educational needs of practicing nurses are so great and so varied. The nature of health care delivery and the direction that nursing moves in the future will have an impact on these educational needs.

Notes

1 Charles H. Judd, "Adult Education," *Amer. J. Nurs.*, 28(7): 654, 1928.

2 Carter V. Good (ed.), *Dictionary of Education*, 2d ed., McGraw-Hill, New York, 1959.

3 *Nursing Thesaurus: A Guide to the Use of Nursing Subject Headings in the International Nursing Index*, 1970-71, p. 5.

4 Op. cit., p. 218.

5 American Nurses' Association, *Facts About Nursing*, The Association, New York, 1968, p. 23.

6 American Nurses' Association, *RNs 1966: An Inventory of Registered Nurses*, The Association, New York, 1969, p. 5.

7 *The Continuing Education Unit: An Interim Statement of the National Task Force to Study the Feasibility and Implementation of a Uniform Unit for the Measurement of Non-Credit Continuing Education Programs*, National University Extension Association, Washington, D.C., n.d. (Mimeographed.)

REFERENCES

American Nurses' Association: *Avenues for Continued Learning*, The Association, New York, 1967.

American Nurses' Association and American Academy of Pediatrics: "Guidelines on Short-Term Continuing Education Programs for Pediatric Nurse Associates," *Amer. J. Nurs.* 71(3): 509-512, 1971.

Andrews, Priscilla M., and Alfred Yankauer: "The Pediatric Nurse Practitioner," *Amer. J. Nurs.*, 71(3): 504-508, 1971.

Aradine, Caroline, and Marc F. Hansen: "Interdisciplinary Teamwork in Family Care: Implications for Clinical Service and Professional Education," *Nurs. Clin. N. Amer.*, 5(2): 111-222, 1970.

Axford, Roger: *Adult Education: The Open Door*, International Textbook Company, Scranton, Pa., 1969, pp. 1-26.

Brown, Clement R., and Henry S. M. Uhl: "Mandatory Continuing Education: Sense or Nonsense?" *J.A.M.A.*, 213(10): 1660-1668, 1970.

Christman, Luther: "Education of the Health Team," *J.A.M.A.*, 213(2): 284-285, 1970.

Conley, Veronica L., and Carol M. Larson: "Among Regional Medical Programs—An Enduring Commitment," *J. Contin. Educ. Nurs.*, 1(4): 28-33, 1970.

Dryden, Virginia: *Nursing Trends*, William C. Brown Publishing Company, Dubuque, Iowa, 1968.

Elkins, Wilson H.: "Education Is Continuous," *Nurs. Outlook*, **9**(4): 243-245, 1961.

Frank, Sister Charles Marie: "On Continuing Growth," *Amer. J. Nurs.*, **60**(10): 1488-1490, 1960.

Gibbs, Getrude E.: "Will Continuing Education Be Required for License Renewal?", *Amer. J. Nurs.*, **71**(11): 2175-2179, 1971.

"Health Maintenance Organizations," *Hospitals, Journal of the American Hospital Association*, **45**(6): 53-81, 1971.

Hornback, May S.: "Continuing Education—Whose Responsibility?" *J. Contin. Educ. Nurs.*, **2**(4): 9-13, 1971.

Hornback, May S. (ed.), "Health Maintenance Organization: Concept and Functions," Conference Proceedings, Department of Nursing, Health Science Unit, University of Wisconsin-Extension, Madison, Wisconsin, 1972.

Hutchison, Dorothy: "Credit for Non-Credit?—An Editorial Exploration," *J. Contin. Educ. Nurs.*, **2**(2): 54-56, 1971.

Kirk, Kenneth W., and Melvin H. Weinswig, "Mandatory Continuing Education for the Relicensure of Pharmacists," *Amer. J. Pharmaceutical Educ.*, **36**(2): 48-55, 1972.

Knowles, Malcolm S.: "Gearing Adult Education for the Seventies," *J. Contin. Educ. Nurs.*, **1**(1): 11-16, 1970.

Komaroff, Anthony L.: "Regional Medical Program in Search of a Mission," *New Eng. J. Med.*, **284**: 758-764, 1971.

Lewis, Edith P. (compiler): *Changing Attitudes of Nursing Practice, New Needs, New Roles*, The American Journal of Nursing Company, New York, 1971.

National Academy of Sciences: *New Members of the Physician's Health Team: Physician's Assistants*, The Academy, Washington, D.C., 1970.

National Commission for the Study of Nursing and Nursing Education: *Nurse Clinician and Physician's Assistant: The Relationship Between Two Emerging Practitioner Concepts*, The Commission, Rochester, N.Y., 1971.

Neylan, Margaret S., et al.: "An Interprofessional Approach to Continuing Education in the Health Sciences," *J. Contin. Educ. Nurs.*, **2**(4): 21-28, 1971.

Nuckolls, Katherine Buckley: "Continuing Education and the Extended Role of the Nurse or the Continuing Role of the Nurse in Extended Education," *J. Contin. Educ. Nurs.*, **2**(4): 29-35, 1971.

Ohliger, John: "Lifelong Learning—Voluntary or Compulsory?" *Adult Lead.*, **17**(3): 124, 1968.

Pelligrino, Edmund D.: "Continuing Education in the Health Professions," *Amer. J. Pharmaceutical Educ.*, **33**(5): 712-720, 1969.

Silver, George A.: "National Health Insurance, National Health Policy, and the National Health," *Amer. J. Nurs.*, **71**(9): 1730-1734, 1971.

Spector, Audrey F.: "The American Nurses' Association and Continuing Education," *J. Contin. Educ. Nurs.*, **2**(2): 41-45, 1971.

2

History of continuing education in nursing

Let us never consider ourselves as finished nurses . . .
We must be learning all of our lives.

—Florence Nightingale

From the above quotation, it is obvious that Florence Nightingale was aware of the need for continuing education for nurses. In spite of this early recognition, the concept of lifelong learning for the practitioner is a relatively recent one. For instance, no reference to continuing education efforts, including postgraduate courses, is made in the index of *American Nursing* by Mary Roberts, published in 1954. This book, a most detailed and definitive history of nursing in the United States, includes only a brief discussion of postgraduate courses. One can conclude that such activity was seen as not particularly important.

Yet the need for continuing education for the practitioner was identified in the first volume of the *American Journal of Nursing.* Urging private duty nurses[1] to add to their store of knowledge by reading, Edith Draper also suggests another source of information: "Those who can would do well to profit by the University Extension courses of lectures now held in almost every city. Half a loaf is better than no bread, and even a few such lectures attentively followed with notes taken would provide some nourishment to a starving mind."[2]

Meetings of various types provided by school of nursing alumnae associations can be considered the first continuing education offerings available to nurses. The programs varied in quality and quantity, but the early graduates attempted to keep informed by participation in these activities.

POSTGRADUATE COURSES

In a paper read in 1901 before the Third Annual Convention of the Nurses' Associated Alumnae of the United States (now the American Nurses' Association), Persis Plumer urged the establishment of postgraduate courses and pointed out that ". . . the advent of medical science, and the changes it brings, makes the nurse a few years back decidedly a back number."[3]

In this paper, the author discussed opportunities to learn on the job: "We lose so many splendid opportunities to learn in the daily struggle with unfamiliar duties in the first months of the hospital! It is so hard to get the work done, we have little or no time to think what it all means, and it is only when the routine has become second nature that we open our eyes to the larger meaning of it all . . ."[4] It hardly seems necessary to add that these comments are as applicable today as when they were first made.

Several articles in the early journals urge the establishment of postgraduate courses; a few authors candidly admit they are badly needed because of the poor instruction in some schools of nursing. It is difficult to determine where the first postgraduate course was offered, but early developments were noted at the Illinois Training School for Nurses in Chicago, where in 1894 a Canadian nurse was accepted for postgraduate training on payment of her expenses. Regular courses for graduate nurses were established in the early 1900s.[5] From these early developments to the present day, many courses have been offered by a wide variety of institutions and agencies.

Postgraduate courses in nursing were usually offered by hospitals, and frequently these courses were designed to provide more knowledge and experience in a specific clinical area. Since there was no educational control of these programs, the amount of instruction varied greatly from one institution to another. All too often there was considerable clinical experience, inadequately supervised, with little theory. In a study conducted for the American Nurses' Association reported in 1929, the hours of instruction ranged from 15 minutes to 15 hours per week.[6] Frequently this aspect of the course consisted of having the nurse attend classes being conducted for undergraduate students. In the absence of educational requirements of the agencies offering the course, the primary purpose most often was to provide nursing service, even though not identified in this way.

Sometimes a fee was charged the nurse enrollee, and in the study reported above, tuition ranged from nothing to $10. It was usually assumed that the nurse paid for the education she received by caring for patients, and frequently she was given a small stipend for this service. It is fair to say that exploitation of these nurses in the name of education was not uncommon, although it is also true that a few truly educational programs were established.

The postgraduate course fell into disfavor in the early 1940s at about the time that increasing numbers of registered nurses began to seek college preparation. Since early postgraduate courses were provided by hospitals and not by institutions of higher learning, enrollees were not awarded college credits. Nurses seeking courses for credit became less interested in participating in the non-college-related program.

Postgraduate courses were offered in many clinical areas: maternity nursing, pediatrics, operating room, psychiatric nursing, communicable disease and tuberculosis nursing. These can more properly be seen as supplemental programs, filling in educational gaps, than as true postgraduate courses. They obviously met a need since many of them existed for some time, and a few remain to the present day.

Postgraduate courses provided the earliest, and for many years almost the only, opportunity for nurses to continue their educations. When courses were well-designed and carefully taught, a good educational experience was provided, and contributed much to nurses' professional knowledge and skills. Postgraduate courses provided a foundation for later developments in continuing education in nursing. Indeed, today's short-term courses in clinical areas bear a strong resemblance to their educational origins.

In the United States the term *postgraduate course* is seldom used in nursing today. In contrast, continuing education courses in medicine are commonly called postgraduate courses, and medical schools often have departments of postgraduate medicine. Nurses may have rejected the designation because the educational soundness of early postgraduate courses for nurses varied. The term became outmoded as it was often associated with apprentice-type nursing education considered by some as inappropriate for the education of professionals.

Lecture Courses

The establishment of lecture courses by alumnae associations of schools of nursing was another early development. Information about these educational pursuits is quite limited; they are mentioned in the early journals, although not in much detail. They usually appeared to be a series of weekly evening lectures, frequently given by a physician, on a variety of clinical subjects. Sociology and psychology were also popular subjects.

Since alumnae frequently stayed in the same community as the school from which they were graduated, the learners were often a closely knit group of nurses, with common interests and common educational backgrounds. In spite of the long arduous work days of early nurses, reports suggest that such sessions were enthusiastically received.

Credit Courses and Summer Programs

The movement of nursing education into the system of higher education, beginning with the courses offered to registered nurses in 1899 at Teachers

College, Columbia University, is closely allied to continuing education efforts. Since this history is related elsewhere, only a few points will be covered here.

In addition to a limited number of formal educational programs leading to a degree, a number of summer programs were offered to nurses in several institutions that had no regular nursing programs. Among the earliest of these offerings was a nursing course given by the University of North Dakota in 1912.[7] This was followed by other university courses; these summer programs were often designed for faculty members of schools of nursing. Some of the offerings carried college credit.

New roles for nurses increased the practitioner's awareness of deficits in educational preparation. The public health nursing role is one illustration; public health nurses were among the first to identify their educational inadequacy. Such recognition in the public health field led to the establishment of specially designed courses. Among the earliest were those offered by Teachers' College, Columbia University, New York; Simmons College, Boston; New Haven Visiting Nurse Association and Yale University; School of Practical Arts, Western Reserve University, Cleveland; School of Civics, Chicago; School of Social Economy, St. Louis.[8] Many of the early courses were established in institutions that did not offer nursing programs, so arrangements were made for affiliation with other schools.

Somewhat unique in its development, the public health nursing course established in Wisconsin in 1916 was a cooperative venture between the Exten-

Figure 2-1   The first class of nurses in the public health nursing course offered in Wisconsin. The course was taught by Katherine Olmsted (seated). (*Photograph courtesy of Susan Normann*)

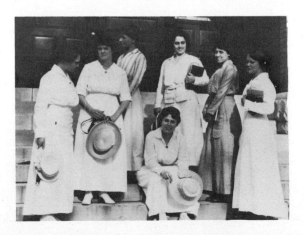

sion Division of the University of Wisconsin and the Wisconsin Anti-Tuberculosis Association (Fig. 2-1). As implied by the sponsorship, much of the early work of the public health nurse was in this area of practice. The eight-week Wisconsin course also focused on the needs of the rural nurse, for the nursing education at the time was not adequate preparation for the responsibilities she faced. Eventually this course was sponsored solely by the Wisconsin Anti-Tuberculosis Association; it continued until 1936, when Marquette University announced the availability of courses for registered nurses.

The short course and summer programs were an attempt to meet the specific educational needs of nurses employed in positions for which they were inadequately prepared. Today we look askance at a nursing course offered by an educational institution without nursing faculty but it is recognized that these courses did contribute to the improvement of nursing education and practice. Perhaps more than anything else they served to whet the enrollee's appetite for more education. This alone is a most significant contribution to the development of nursing as a profession.

INSTITUTES, WORKSHOPS AND CONFERENCES

The first reference to institutes designed for nurses appeared in the *American Journal of Nursing* in the early 1920s. Many of the early institutes were sponsored by the American Nurses' Association, the National League of Nursing Education (NLNE), or their state or local affiliates. Others were offered through colleges and universities. Many of the early institutes, particularly those sponsored by the NLNE, were planned for teachers of nursing. Institutes designed for other groups reflected various nurses' occupational learning needs, and were identified by such titles as: "Tuberculosis Nursing," "The Modern Health Movement," "Supervision of Nurses in Training."

The short-term course, by whatever title it is known, can contribute to improved nursing care. Today, courses for nurses are sponsored by many groups: colleges and universities, nursing organizations, health-related organizations of many types, medical societies, state and local health departments. Many of these efforts are sporadic and unrelated and their total impact is questionable. The need for coordination of programs is apparent.

REFRESHER COURSE FOR INACTIVE NURSES

The earliest references to refresher courses for inactive nurses appear in the nursing literature of the early 1930s. The courses were suggested as a means of helping nurses keep updated and of occupying their time during periods of enforced leisure resulting from unemployment. Courses were often sponsored by district nurses' associations.

Interest in the inactive nurse has been greatest during periods of crisis. Shortly before the United States entered World War II, refresher courses were offered by several different groups. Frequently schools of nursing sponsored courses primarily designed for their alumni. Reports on school-related refresher courses appear in the nursing literature beginning in 1940.

The first reported statewide program for inactive nurses was that offered in 1941 in New York through the State League for Nursing Education. About the same time, a statewide program was launched in Michigan, coordinated through the Extension Service of the University of Michigan, in cooperation with Wayne University (now Wayne State University) in Detroit. The faculty, directed by Thelma Brewington, included three full-time instructors. Statewide planning was also done in Washington, where courses were offered through the Extension Service of the University of Washington.

The first federal legislation for the support of nursing education included provisions for refresher courses for inactive nurses, in addition to funds for basic and advanced nursing education. Public Law 146 (77th Congress), titled "Training for Nurses (National Defense)" was passed July 1, 1941, and funds were allocated the following March. One hundred one programs for inactive nurses were conducted during 1942-1943, and over 3,000 enrollees completed the course.[9]

The Bolton Nursing Training Act, Public Law 74 (78th Congress), was passed on July 15, 1943; it is most familiar as the legislation creating the Cadet Nurse Corps, but it also included provisions for courses for inactive nurses. However, the need for these courses was apparently met through allocations provided by the previous act, since no courses for inactive nurses were offered through the Bolton Act.

Following World War II, interest in inactive nurses was sporadic until about 1950, when these nurses began to be viewed as a source of supply in the face of an ever-increasing shortage of nursing personnel.

Recent Developments

Funds for refresher courses for inactive nurses are now available in certain areas under the provisions of the Manpower Development and Training Act of 1962. This legislation was designed primarily to retain workers who became unemployed through automation, but inactive nurses may qualify for special courses designed to update their nursing skills.

In June 1967 federal funds became available to launch a nationwide program designed to facilitate the return of the inactive nurse to practice. Contracts between states and the Division of Nursing in the Public Health Service, U.S. Department of Health, Education and Welfare, provided funds for the employment of a state coordinator and for other administrative costs. One-year contracts were granted to forty-six agencies, usually state nurses' associations or health departments, but a few contracts were with state universities. Most of the contracts were extended beyond the first year.

One thousand eight refresher courses were offered to inactive nurses between July 1967 and August 1970; of these courses, 458 were funded through the Manpower Development and Training Act. In this period of time, 11,455 inactive nurses completed refresher courses.[10] It is too soon to evaluate the total effects of this effort, but the federally funded project appears to have achieved its purpose: the return of the inactive nurse to practice.

Refresher courses are discussed in more detail in Chapter 10. This brief review not only provides historical background, but suggests that the need for some type of continuing education for inactive nurses is an ongoing one.

IN-SERVICE EDUCATION

Much of the early writing about in-service education is identified in the nursing literature by the words *staff education.* As with other early developments in nursing, it is difficult to pinpoint the early history of in-service education, since those involved rarely wrote about their experiences. Also, it is sometimes difficult to separate staff education from postgraduate courses offered by a particular institution. Obviously, learning on the job is as old as nursing itself, but early efforts at some type of organized learning approaches were not described in the nursing literature.

In discussing early developments, Blanche Pfefferkorn writes, "No printed record has been found of definite programs of staff education for the hospital and nursing school staff, but that such programs do exist, we know. Many institutions hold regular faculty conferences and in a number of instances a program is carefully worked out."[11]

Education for staff nurses provided by the employing agency (though frequently on the nurse's off-duty time) is first discussed in the nursing periodicals in 1929, and articles on the subject occur at intervals during the next decade. These articles often include descriptions of the content of the programs offered by a particular institution.

Early efforts at staff education in hospitals parallel rather closely the efforts to upgrade teachers in the public school system through the provision of in-service training. A later impetus to the development of education provided by the employing agency follows the pattern of on-the-job training established in industry particularly during and immediately following World War II.

One of the earliest descriptions of an in-service education program to appear in the nursing literature was that offered under the auspices of the Illinois Training School in Chicago. This program, described in 1929, was designed for the staff of Cook County Hospital; not only were supervisors, head nurses, and general duty nurses included, but a special program was also planned for the attendants employed by the hospital. In describing the program Katharine Densford gives a word of warning which is as applicable today as when it was first noted: "Not until we have proper care, properly given, in our hospital units can we expect our staff education program to attain maximum, or even moderate efficiency."[12]

Credit for the idea of the staff education program at Cook County Hospital is given to Laura Logan, dean of the Illinois Training School, who provided the climate and leadership for the development of all programs. Much of the planning, direction, and coordination for the program was the responsibility of Katharine Densford, then serving as Miss Logan's first assistant.[13] Perhaps one of the earliest credit courses to be given on the subject of in-service education was that offered by the University of Minnesota in 1955, during Miss Densford's tenure as dean of that school of nursing. The provision of this course no doubt reflected her continued interest in in-service education.

Another early development took place in Veteran's Administration hospitals. Initially programs were planned for all nurses who had no education or experience in psychiatric nursing, but content later also included tuberculosis nursing. Since this education was provided to nurses employed in the institution, it can properly be seen as in-service education; since it appears to have served the purpose of filling education gaps in the basic nursing program, it might also be considered postgraduate training.

Early staff education programs for practicing nurses often were primarily lectures by physicians. Additional content included reviewing nursing procedures, learning to operate new equipment, and studying the policies of the institution. Infrequently, staff nurses were asked for their suggestions for program content; questionnaires were sometimes distributed to elicit this information.

From these early developments, the concept of in-service education for practicing nurses slowly evolved in hospitals and other health agencies. This snail's pace development can be attributed to many underlying reasons: failure of nurses to recognize their own learning needs; lack of administrative and budgetary support; difficulty in measuring learning outcome, particularly that relating to improved nursing care; fading interest of nurses as the result of ineffective programs.

There seems little doubt that the ineffectiveness of many in-service programs resulted from the inadequate preparation of the nursing staff responsible for the program. Many hospitals appear to have established in-service programs because it was the thing to do, without careful consideration of the many factors involved in providing an effective program.

Training of Nursing Assistants

The exigencies of World War II led to the development of the nursing assistant as we know him today. The success of the volunteer Red Cross nurses' aide in civilian hospitals and the medical corpsman in military hospitals were both influential in promoting the use of this worker. Once this employee found a place in the hospital setting, numbers rapidly increased.

Nursing aides were used during World War I, and during the depression of the 1930s, housekeeping aides were employed in many governmental hospitals. These trained ward helpers were employed through the federal Works Projects Administration (WPA) whose projects were designed to employ people in an economy where jobs were scarce. These were significant developments in the history of the use of auxiliary personnel, but did not have the impact of the use of civilian and military aides during World War II.

The training and use of these employees in the 1940s was haphazard and disorganized. Although some institutions applied the principles followed in the Training Within Industry (TWI) program, for the most part the aide learned his job by working with another aide, rather than through an organized training program.

The use of auxiliary workers in hospitals expanded rapidly following World War II. This rapid expansion and the new workers' lack of adequate preparation for their job responsibilities generated concern, as was voiced in 1952 by the Joint Commission for the Improvement of the Care of the Patient. This group, made up of representatives of the American Hospital Association, American Medical Association, and the American Nurses' Association, made a formal recommendation that each institution employing nonprofessional personnel conduct well-planned on-the-job training programs for these employees.

Two years later, a nationwide Nursing Aide In-service Training Project was launched to implement the recommendation. This project was cosponsored by the American Hospital Association, National League for Nursing, and the U.S. Public Health Service. Training auxiliary workers required trained teachers, and to meet this need, the Department of Hospital Nursing of the NLN planned regional teacher-trainer institutes.

A pilot project was set up for the Maryland, Delaware, and Washington, D.C. area in January 1954. Following this successful trial, five-day regional institutes were offered to nurse teachers throughout the country. Using a multiplier method of instruction, the teacher-trainers returned to their communities and taught professional nurses who were directing auxiliary nursing personnel.

All but thirteen states in the country participated in the project. By August 1954, twenty-seven regional institutes were held, with 246 teacher-trainers participating. These teachers in turn, conducted 480 workshops attended by 3,522 instructors from hospitals and nursing homes.[14]

The evaluation of this extensive program indicated that it met a serious educational need, and also that it had a significant impact on the quality of care provided by participating institutions. In discussing this development, a landmark document must be mentioned. It is the *Handbook for Nursing Aides in Hospitals*, and the accompanying instructor's manual, developed by the U.S.

Public Health Service and published by the American Hospital Association in 1953. This publication gave formal recognition to the types of tasks that could be safely performed by adequately trained auxiliary personnel, and helped establish a consistency in training programs.

A more recent development is the provision of preservice training programs for nursing assistants by increasing numbers of vocational schools. This removes the responsibility for the initial training of these workers from the employing institution, but does not lessen its responsibility for an adequate orientation and continued in-service education when the assistant has been hired.

Organization of In-Service Education

Today, in-service education is seen as an integral part of an effective nursing service, but this has been a slow development. Emory University Hospitals in Atlanta established a separate division of in-service education in the nursing service department in 1952, and other institutions soon adopted this pattern. New patterns of organization are now emerging within institutions, but the agency's responsibility for providing its employees with opportunities for learning has been firmly established. Nursing may be only one aspect of the hospital's ongoing training and development program, but since nursing personnel comprise by far the largest percentage of the hospital's employees, the special importance of the nursing in-service education program is apparent.

As nursing becomes ever more complex, and as nurses, along with the rest of the nation's population, become more mobile, the demand for effective orientation and staff development programs becomes more urgent. Establishing more effective programs is discussed in detail in Chapter 11.

UNIVERSITY INVOLVEMENT IN CONTINUING EDUCATION FOR NURSES

As suggested earlier, initial involvement of universities in continuing education for nurses began in the early 1920s. This interest was sporadic until 1959 when federal funds became available for short-term courses. However, some earlier developments are worth noting.

Occasionally, credit and noncredit courses for nurses were offered in various parts of the country, often under the auspices of the extension division of a university. Pioneering institutions in this endeavor included the University of Pennsylvania, the University of Washington, the University of Pittsburgh. Such courses were provided at the University of Wisconsin before its school of nursing was established, and this may have been true in others.

The courses offered by colleges and universities varied from one- or two-day workshops to classes held weekly for an entire quarter or semester.

Content varied, but a number of the courses were related to functional areas of nursing, such as supervision or ward administration.

The University of Wisconsin appears to have been the first university to appoint a faculty member whose major responsibility was continuing education in nursing. In 1955 a department of nursing was created in the extension division of that university; it was established to provide continuing education opportunities to nurses throughout the state. This was followed shortly by a similar development at the University of Michigan, where a faculty member was appointed jointly to the school of nursing and the extension service.

In 1957 the W. K. Kellogg Foundation funded an experimental program for registered nurses in administrative and teaching positions. Three western institutions, the University of Washington, the University of Colorado, and the University of California in Los Angeles, participated in the three-year program, which consisted of five-day conferences held three times a year.

The year 1957 also saw the beginning of the Western Council on Higher Education for Nursing (WCHEN), established as one of the councils of the Western Interstate Commission of Higher Education, founded in 1951 by the governors of the eleven western states (Alaska and Hawaii joined later). WCHEN established a pattern for interstate planning and cooperation in nursing, including continuing education, and has had a significant impact on the development of such efforts.

The acceptance by university schools of nursing of their responsibility for the continuing education of nurses has evolved slowly. Many of the schools are beset by problems relating to undergraduate education: insufficient funds, inadequate numbers of faculty, poorly prepared faculty, large numbers of students. In the face of these obstacles, a lack of enthusiasm for continuing education is understandable.

In 1967 an attempt was made to provide an opportunity for nursing faculty involved in continuing education to meet at the University of Wisconsin; this meeting was cancelled because of insufficient enrollment. In March 1968 a national conference on continuing education in nursing was held at the University of Wisconsin with thirty-four enrollees; this conference followed a meeting held for nurses involved in regional medical programs. In November of the next year over 100 enrollees attended a conference on continuing education in nursing sponsored by the Medical College of Virginia, Virginia Commonwealth University and held in Williamsburg. The increasing interest and involvement of nurses in continuing education is apparent in these developments.

In recent years a large number of universities with collegiate schools of nursing have appointed faculty members for continuing education programs. Frequently this is not the individual's only assignment, but is a recognition by the university of its responsibility for continuing education of nurses. The role of the university in continuing education will be considered from a broad perspective in the next chapter.

FEDERAL SUPPORT OF CONTINUING EDUCATION

The Social Security Act of 1935 was the first federal legislation to include funds for continuing education of nurses. Under the provisions of this legislation, stipends were available for the preparation of public health nurses. By 1940 approximately 3,000 registered nurses received financial assistance from Social Security funds for some type of preparation in public health nursing.[15] Financial support for refresher courses for inactive nurses is discussed on p. 24.

Later legislation, the Health Amendments Act of 1956, provided a greater impact on continuing education in nursing. The act provided for education of professional nurses in public health, administrative, supervisory, and teaching positions. Grants were made to institutions of higher learning, which in turn awarded traineeships to individual applicants. The legislation enabled many nurses to complete requirements for a baccalaureate degree, and others to secure graduate education.

Initially these funds were designed only for nurses enrolled full-time in college courses. In 1959 the legislation was amended to permit the use of funds to provide tuition and living expenses for nurses enrolled in short-term courses.

Provisions for short-term courses were included in the Nurse Training Act of 1964, which permitted a continuation of educational benefits for nurses. Federal support for nursing education, including short-term courses, were continued in the Health Manpower Act of 1968.

Federal funding for short-term courses came at a time when individual nurses were recognizing their own need for continuing their education. The support enabled many educational institutions and other agencies, such as health departments, to provide needed courses to practicing nurses. Without financial assistance, continuing education programs in nursing would have developed much more slowly.

Federal funds not designed primarily for nurses have also supported continuing education programs in nursing. In a few states, courses were offered through the provisions of Title I of the Higher Education Act of 1965.

Nursing is frequently included in regional medical programs, which were created under Public Law 89-239, passed in 1965. A number of intensive coronary care courses were funded through these programs. In many areas of the country, intensive short-term training courses in a wide variety of content areas were made available to nurses for the first time. The programs permitted the development and use of new media, such as the telephone Dial Access system inaugurated in Wisconsin (Figs. 2-2A and 2-2B).

INTERNATIONAL DEVELOPMENTS

A history of continuing education in nursing would not be complete without some reference to international developments. Space permits a discussion of only a few of these activities.

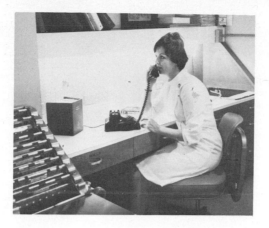

Figure 2-2A A telephone dial-access system provides easy access to
nursing information and is especially valuable to the nurse
who works alone, as on night
duty. (*Gary Schulz, University of Wisconsin Extension*)

The need for additional educational preparation, particularly in public
health nursing, was identified by many nurses working with the League of Red
Cross Societies in the war-torn countries of Europe immediately following World
War I. Organized through the auspices of the League of Red Cross Societies, a
course in public health nursing was established in 1920 at King's College for
Women at the University of London and transferred to Bedford College a year
later. A course designed for nurse administrators and teachers was established in
1924.

Nurses from all over the world attended these year-long programs. By
1933, over 200 nurses from forty-one different countries had completed the
courses.

Originally scholarship assistance was provided by the League of Red Cross
Societies. In 1934 the Florence Nightingale International Foundation established
an endowed trust to provide financial assistance to nurses wishing additional
education, permitting the Bedford College program to continue until it was
interrupted by the war in 1939. Funds for postgraduate nursing education were
later continued, and nurses could choose to attend courses offered in other
countries.

The program offered at Bedford College has had a significant impact on
nursing around the world as a unique opportunity for nurses to add to their
formal education. Alumnae, organized in 1925 as the "Old Internationals," were

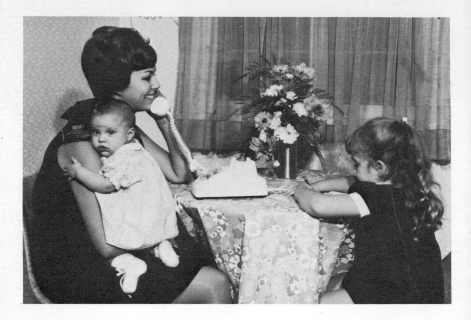

Figure 2-2B   Another advantage in the telephone dial access system
is its availability from any telephone. Here the nurse
calls from her home telephone. (*Gary Schulz, University
of Wisconsin Extension*)

the nursing leaders in their own countries, and influenced international developments in nursing as well.

In August 1964, seventy-eight nurses from nineteen different countries
attended a ten-day conference held at the University of Edinburgh in Scotland.
Although titled an Old Internationals conference, over half of those participating
did not belong to that elite group of nurses. This international workshop
provided an opportunity for nurses from various parts of the world to meet and
study together. Though not the first international nursing conference, it was
unique in that the nurses who attended came not by special invitation, but by
their own expressed interest. Four years later a second conference was held in
Athens, and future conferences are anticipated.

Significant continuing education programs are now conducted in many
parts of the world. Some of these efforts have been sponsored by the World
Health Organization or the International Council of Nurses. When the Four-

teenth Quadrennial Congress of the International Council of Nurses met in Montreal, Canada in June 1969, a concurrent session was planned for nurses involved in programs of continuing education. The idea for this half-day session came from Margaret Neylan, who is responsible for the continuing education program at the University of British Columbia in Vancouver, and the program was presented at McGill University. Continuing education was not seen as a topic significant enough for the regular program of the Congress, but the nurses who attended the half-day session must surely have felt the historic import of the meeting: this was the first international conference on continuing nursing education.

Other Developments

Nurses in many countries are involved in continuing education efforts, but only two such efforts will be discussed here. The first of these is the Royal College of Nursing in Great Britain.

The College of Nursing was founded in 1916 as an organization analagous to the College of Physicians and Surgeons; the title was changed to the Royal College of Nursing by King George in 1939. Among its several purposes is the promotion of nursing education and the advancement of nursing as a profession. Thus it can be seen as an organizational counterpart of the American Nurses' Association.

In 1930 a separate education department was created in the College and within four years this department was established as a national and international center for postcertificate nursing education. An industrial nursing course was started as early as 1934; others were added as the need arose: a nurse teacher's course, a program for health visitors and district nursing, one in nursing administration.

Since nursing is not generally accepted as an educational discipline in nearly all of the institutions of higher learning in Great Britain, the educational program of the Royal College of Nursing was particularly significant. The College continues to meet this educational need to the present day.

One Canadian effort will be noted, since this is a slightly different approach to continuing nursing education. In 1961 a correspondence course in nursing unit administration was developed cooperatively by the Canadian Nurses' Association and the Canadian Hospital Association, with financial support from the W. K. Kellogg Foundation. The course was designed to assist head nurses who were unable to attend regular university programs to upgrade their skills in the administration of hospital nursing units. This course is described in more detail in Chapter 12.

Significant efforts in continuing education are being made by nurses in many other countries of the world. These are frequently identified in international nursing publications.

SUMMARY

The idea of continuing education in nursing is as old as organized nursing, but the concept of lifelong learning for the practitioner has developed slowly. Nevertheless, many educational efforts can be identified as continuing education for practicing nurses.

The history of continuing education in nursing has shown that educational institutions generally have been slow to accept responsibility for assisting the practitioner who wishes to add to her nursing knowledge and skill. If the patterns of nursing education follow general education, it can be predicted that this process will be reversed in the future.

Notes

1. It is helpful to recall that the great majority of nurses practicing at the turn of the century were private duty nurses.

2. Edith A. Draper, "The Value of General Reading for Private Duty Nurses," *Amer. J. Nurs.*, 1(2):205-208, 1901.

3. Persis Plumer, "The Necessity for the Development of Post-Graduate Work," *Amer. J. Nurs.*, 1(10):754, 1901.

4. Ibid., p. 756.

5. Grace Fay Schryver, *A History of the Illinois Training School for Nurses 1880-1929*, Board of Directors of the Illinois Training School for Nurses, Chicago, 1930.

6. Caroline Gray, "Postgraduate Courses," *Amer. J. Nurs.*, 29(6):709, 1929.

7. Blanche Pfefferkorn, "Improvement of the Nurse in Service: An Historical Review," *Amer. J. Nurs.*, 28(7):705, 1928.

8. "Courses in Public Health Nursing," *Public Health Reports*, 34(23):1270, 1919.

9. U.S. Public Health Service, *Annual Report for the Fiscal Years 1941-42; 1942-43*, U.S. Government Printing Office, Washington, D.C., 1950, p. 170.

10. Information from Mrs. Margaret Sheehan, Division of Nursing, Department of Health, Education and Welfare. Statistics do not include the state of Michigan.

11. Blanche Pfefferkorn, "Improvement of the Nurse in Service: An Historical Review," *Amer. J. Nurs.*, 28(7):709, 1928.

12. Katharine Densford: "An 'In-Service' Program of Staff Education," *Thirty Fifth Annual Report, National League of Nursing Education*, 1929, p. 117.

13. Personal correspondence with Katharine Densford Dreves, March 7, 1970.

14. Margaret Giffin, "Teaching by the Thousands," *Nurs. Outlook*, 4(8):462, 1956.

15. Mary M. Roberts, *American Nursing: History and Interpretation*, The Macmillan Company, New York, 1954, p. 274.

REFERENCES

Beck, Sister Berenice: "Staff Education Programs," *Amer. J. Nurs.*, **34**(9):901-907, 1934.

Bowman, Gerald: *The Lamp and the Book: The Story of the RCN, 1916-1966,* The Queen Anne Press, Limited, London, 1967.

Carter, Maynard: "International Courses at Bedford College, University of London," *The I.C.N.*, **3**:25-29, 1928.

Cooper, Signe S.: "Activating the Inactive Nurse: A Historical Review," *Nurs. Outlook*, **15**(10):62-65, 1967.

————: "University Extension Courses for Nurses," *Nurs. Outlook,* **11**(1) 36-39, 1963.

Coulter, Pearl Parvin: "Continuing Education for Nurses in the West," *Nurs. Outlook,* **10**(2): 113-117, 1962.

Densford, Katharine J.: "Staff Education," *Amer. J. Nurs.*, **29**(10): 1239-1246, 1929.

Germain, Lucy: "Continuing In-Service Education," *Amer. J. Nurs.*, **51**(11):670-672, 1951.

Giffin, Margaret: "Teaching by the Thousands," *Nurs. Outlook*, **4**(8):460-463, 1956.

Judd, Charles H.: "Adult Education," *Amer. J. Nurs.*, **28**(7):654-656, 1928.

Kuehn, Ruth Perkins: "Continuing Education in Nursing," *J.A.M.A.* **190**(6): 544-545, 1964.

McClaskie, Maude: "Postgraduate Work," *American Society of Superintendents of Training Schools, Ninth Annual Report*, 1902, pp. 90-93.

McManus, R. Louise: "What Colleges and Universities Offer the Practicing Nurse," *Amer. J. Nurs.*, **54**(12):1478-80, 1954.

Niles, Anne McKee: "Call Nursing Dial Access," *Amer. J. Nurs.*, **69**(6):1235-1236, 1969.

Pfefferkorn, Blanche: "Improvement of the Nurse in Service: An Historical Review," *Amer. J. Nurs.*, **28**(7):700-710, 1928.

Poole, Drusilla: "Inservice Education Reaches a Milestone," *Amer. J. Nurs.*, **53**(12): 1456-1459, 1953.

Proceedings Conference on Continuing Nursing Education held June 24, 1969, The University of British Columbia, Vancouver, n.d. (Mimeographed).

Report of the Old Internationals Summer School, August, 1964, D. J. Jeffery, Ltd., Harpenden, England, n.d.

Roberts, Mary M.: *American Nursing: History and Interpretation*, The Macmillan Company, New York, 1954.

Smith, Harriet: "An Experiment in Continuing Education in Nursing," *Int. Nurs. Rev.*, **15**(2): 134-140, 1968.

Stewart, Isabel: "Postgraduate Education—Old and New," *Amer. J. Nurs.*, **33**(4):361-369, 1933.

————: "Summer Institutes for Superintendents and Teachers of Nursing Schools," *Amer. J. Nurs.*, **20**(7):549-551, 1920.

3

Trends in adult education

BURTON W. KREITLOW

Professor of Adult Education
University of Wisconsin
Madison, Wisconsin

The roots of adult education are hidden in man's primitive past. Thus, to examine trends in adult education one must look back as well as ahead. In this chapter this will be done first, by a broad sweep of the history of adult education and second, by an assessment and identification of current trends and a view toward the future.

HISTORY

The use of drawings on cave walls to pass concepts from one generation to the next could be identified as one of the earliest examples of a program in adult education. So, too, could the intensive training that was given by one shaman or medicine man to a novice as he learned to bargain with the spiritual world. It is more relevant, however, to identify the roots of adult education with first written records of the Sumerians at about 3000 B.C. From wherever come our first examples of adult education it is realistic to begin in pre-Christian times. From then on needs for continued learning can be identified and the invention of programs for continued learning can be viewed from century to century. As is the case with many other historical developments, adult education has made startling growth in the past two centuries.

We may look to ancient Egypt to find the first examples of a highly specialized society with technical training developed for its artisans and priestly class. Egyptian wisdom was embodied in many myths with the interpretation of these in the hands of the priests. Physicians were trained through a program of apprenticeships not far removed in principle from those which followed through the centuries in this and other fields. The development of a university at Alexandria was a timely innovation in adult education and the libraries, botanical gardens, zoological and medical facilities that were open to the right adults were precursors of institutions that were to follow many centuries later.

A model for the organization for training the masses can be found in the Hebrew culture. Synagogues were originally based upon the concept of education in the neighborhood. Although the subject matter was predominantly religious in nature, some part of this early education was designed for the purposes of health.

Greek society was the first to establish moral excellence as a goal of education. The militant arete was involved in an adult training program in the use of arms. From this beginning the military has provided an example of a highly structured and objectively focused adult education program. The roots of physical education training for adults was embodied in the gymnasiums of early Greece. These were much like programs for young adults in the YMCAs and YWCAs of today. Traveling sophists taught rhetoric and politics and Socrates talked to any and all who would stop and listen. As one of the first great teachers, Socrates dealt almost exclusively with the adult population. Plato advocated adult education and strongly supported education as a lifelong process.

Roman civilization continued much of the Greek and Egyptian traditions. Libraries were established, traveling rhetoricians moved about the country, speaking on subjects of concern in that day. This was a means for bringing new ideas from the center of civilization to the hinterland as the precursor of a modern extension system. If today, someone were asked where the concept of extension began a reference to nineteenth century developments in the United States would be expected, yet the concept is far older than this. The most extensive early extension effort was not called extension, but was led by Christ, his disciples, and followers who organized neighborhoods, cities, counties, states and countries in an effort to carry the Word through the known world.

Yet five hundred years earlier, a less well organized but similar system of extension was developed in a totally different culture, China. Here Confucius, at the age of 22, had become a well known teacher and noted people were gathering at his house for interpretation of ideas on practical morality and the deeds of man in relation to his fellowmen. Then he likewise, along with his disciples, traveled far and wide spreading his concepts of practical morality.

The next big surge in adult education came with the information distribution impact provided by printing in the fifteenth century. Although its initial focus was religious in nature, it provided the base upon which libraries could be developed in earnest. Science began to redevelop following its decline during the dark ages and the new technology provided for a communications acceleration with new potential. Seventeenth- and eighteenth-century innovations in England provided the pool from which many ideas were borrowed by the American colonies as they established their first adult education programs. These were largely programs with a religious orientation using and developing limited resources for educational purposes. The Society for the Propagation of Christian Knowledge had literacy as its major goal in order that adults could read the Bible. These programs also had goals encouraging adults to better accept their lot, to be more efficient producers, to be temperate, clean and honest. This puritan influence crossed the Atlantic to the developing Americas where Cotton Mather in Massachusetts in 1710 published *Essays To Do Good* advocating neighborhood discussion groups which would aid in the preservation of puritanical values. This may have been the first written proposal for adult education in America and included such subjects as religion, politics and ideas for advancing the society.

The American colonies were also inventing their own forms of adult education. In 1727 Benjamin Franklin proposed the Junto, where subject matter was to include morals, politics, and science and where members were to produce essays for discussion. Poor Richard's Almanac was a creation of this remarkable man, again with an objective of spreading information to the remote parts. A study of Franklin suggests that he initiated more innovations and modifications in adult education methods, theory, and subject matter than any person before or since.

The colonies, and later the United States, continued borrowing from England and the rest of Europe. John Wesley, the Methodist theologian and "extension man," demonstrated by his travels in Britain how he could influence local congregations. This practice was copied in the new states. Classes for literacy were begun in order that more people might have access to the Bible. Pamphlets written by Wesley were reprinted and widely disseminated in the United States. In 1814 Denmark became the first country to establish state support for adult education and later developed widespread evening classes as part of that program. The folk high schools were founded to provide a place of learning during the long winter months and programmed for both practical matters and cultural nationalism. Mechanic institutes first organized in England in the 1820s were focused on the promotion of knowledge that was behind the trades, drawing, geography, morals and history. Almost immediately this idea was transferred to Boston where Timothy Claxton organized a mechanics institute and gave popular lectures on science.

The last half of the nineteenth century saw the development of the real base for the modern era of adult education in the United States. It is not important to identify one particular program most significant in this development but the national government's recognition that adult education was worthy of financial support was a cornerstone. The Morrill Act of 1862, which established the land grant colleges, demonstrated this commitment. So too did the Hatch Act of 1887, which established experiment stations. Likewise, the acceptance of the adult education concept in the 1880s by institutions of higher

---

Exhibit 3.1 HISTORICAL EVOLUTION OF ADULT EDUCATION

I. Early Beginnings

1. Learning to survive
2. Development in early civilizations (Sumerian, Assyrian, Egyptian, Chinese, Greek, and Roman)
3. Religious education in the Christian era
4. Islamic civilization and the diffusion of knowledge

II. Colonial America

1. Jamestown—1607
2. Harvard University—1636
3. Junto discussion club—1730
4. Subscription library—1735
5. Massachusetts Historical Society Museum—1790

III. United States—19th Century

1. Pennsylvania Academy of Fine Arts—1805
2. Mechanics and mercantile libraries and institutes—1831
3. Lyceum movement—1826
4. Popular reading and free public libraries—1852
5. Evening schools—1810
6. Government support and programming for adult education on national scale—1887
7. Higher education and adult education—1880

IV. 20th Century and Modern Era

1. Post-World War I idealism and great optimism (1919-1929)
2. Period of social, economic, and political crisis (1930-1946)
3. Professionalization and institutionalization of adult education (1947 to present)

education in Wisconsin, Minnesota and California helped launch the modern era. Because of these pioneering actions, a number of the institutions were ready when the time for rapid development of adult and continuing education came.

Webster Cotton suggests that the modern era begins in 1919.[1] I believe it began somewhat earlier than that but will accept Cotton's format as a reasonable one. Certainly aspects of the modern era had arrived with the establishment of the Cooperative Extension Service before World War I. With this act, adult education began the move from content to problem solving. However, the revitalization of adult education was post-World War I. With the input of the Carnegie Corporation in 1925, with the writings of Eduard C. Lindemann in the 1920s and the social reformists, Laski, Hart, and Kilpatrick, continuing education was recognized as a necessary part of modern life.

It was in the 1920s and 1930s that the professionalization and organization for adult continuing education began in earnest. In 1926 the American Association for Adult Education was founded; in 1929 the Journal of Adult Education. In 1935 the first Ph.D. degree in adult education was granted at Teachers College, Columbia University. The first textbook organized for adult education classes was written by Lyman Bryson in 1936. These actions were moving adult education from the periphery of other fields to the establishment of adult education as a special field of its own. The American Association for Adult Education disbanded and the new Adult Education Association of the U.S.A. came into being in 1951. The Ford Foundation and the Kellogg Foundation stimulated a new professionalism. Adult education was finding its place and playing a new and significant role in the educational programs of American society. In Exhibit 3.1 an outline (from a combination of materials found primarily in the writings of Liveright,[2] Cotton,[3] and Knowles[4]) summarizes this historical evolution for the United States.

Exhibit 3.2 shows in simple diagram form the development of adult education in perspective from its roots to its major developments in Europe and up to the modern era. A person interested in the continuing education in any of the health fields would find it challenging to take a historical view of adult education in his own specialty.

CURRENT TRENDS

Acceptance of Continued Learning

The Johnstone study pointed out that in 1962 over 24 million adults participated in adult education programs. The more recent investigation of adult learning projects by Tough[5] would indicate that if the individual projects of each adult were identified the Johnstone figures would be more than doubled as of 1972. Learning has been accepted as a part of life by a very large proportion of

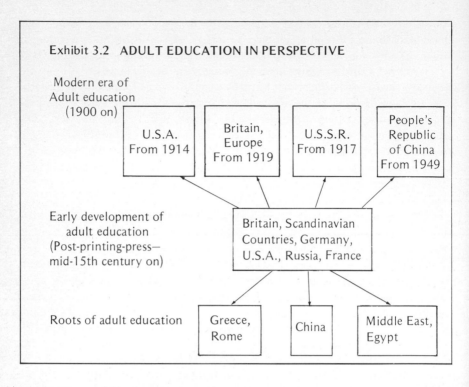

Exhibit 3.2 ADULT EDUCATION IN PERSPECTIVE

Modern era of
Adult education
(1900 on)

| U.S.A. From 1914 | Britain, Europe From 1919 | U.S.S.R. From 1917 | People's Republic of China From 1949 |

Early development of
adult education
(Post-printing-press—
mid-15th century on)

Britain, Scandinavian Countries, Germany, U.S.A., Russia, France

Roots of adult education

| Greece, Rome | China | Middle East, Egypt |

the adults in American society. Much of this may be related to the changes in technology, in professionalism, and in urbanization. It is clear from research that education begets education. For example, the person with schooling beyond a college degree participates more in continuing education than the person with the college degree. A person with a college degree participates more than the person with a high school education. A person who is a high school graduate participates more in continuing education than the person who never attended high school. As the level of education has been raised in the United States, the recognition of the need for continuing education has risen along with it.

Number and Characteristics of Participants

Over twenty-four million adults participate in organized adult education programs. There are millions more involved in their own learning programs and each year shows an increasing participation in many existing programs and new programs are begun.

The emergence of Adult Basic Education programs (ABE) in the mid-sixties was responsible for the development of an almost totally new group of participants among those of low literacy. Although this program borrowed much from the early Americanization programs of the 1920s it was dealing with the considerably different cultural mix than the earlier program developed for new immigrants. The ABE program began to deal with those whose education had been thwarted by certain characteristics of American society. It sought students from among the disadvantaged, among those against whom prejudice was more than spoken, from those in isolated areas and from the migrants in the seasonal migrant streams. Thus, today each state has a program for Adult Basic Education while in 1960 there were very few.

The sheer increase in the level of education and the extent to which young adults have continued their education beyond college graduation has created an inherent pressure toward more participation in adult learning activities. Participation in adult programs by new college graduates, by those who have continued on toward master's and even doctor's degrees have increased.

The number of young adults showing up in programs sponsored by libraries, YMCAs and YWCAs, extension services, and public schools and in special government education programs has been especially noted when the focus is on social improvement.

There have been new and continuing efforts to reach adults in the upper age brackets as society has recognized the proportionate increase in their numbers. No extensive participation increase from this group has yet been noted but the basis for an increase is real.

Nature of the Programs

An overview of what is being offered and of the needs being responded to by adult education agencies is mind-boggling. As of this point of time in the United States there is more comprehensive planning for adult education than at any time in history. More agencies are looking at the needs of particular clientele groups. More specialists are pointing out those aspects of their field that are needed to survive in present society. Adult education agencies are being more specific in terms of their own goals, philosophies, and purposes, and adults are beginning to spell out their needs more specifically and more vocally. Programs are becoming broader and more comprehensive. For example, certain formalized vocational adult programs are, in fact, becoming programs toward associate degrees where some of the work taken in the vocational program is transferrable as college credit to other institutions of higher learning. At the same time that this is occurring there are programs that are less formal in class organization and teaching. The range of opportunity widens, and as before, in response to the changing nature of society. In this instance a demand for learner input into goal setting and program format brings personalized goals and creative self-instruction.

Changing work patterns have increased the possibility of residential adult education. Throughout the United States on any weekend there are thousands of residential conferences meeting in special centers, in hotels, in motels, in special campus facilities, on-campus and in campus residential centers away from the mainstream of modern life.

Professional organizations for teachers, pharmacists, nurses, and attorneys have sought and are getting more in-service programs to develop a greater competency in the day to day operation of their jobs.

At the same time individuals are finding more and more opportunity for independent study made possible by the vast increase of communication resources from paperback books to expanded library services, to articulated instructional media from universities and through special efforts by national education television and radio, to meet needs of modern man.

Adult education during the decade of the sixties became broader on the one hand and provided more opportunity for more depth on the other. There were programs for the illiterates and programs for the philosopher. There were programs on executive management and programs in the cultural arts. Throughout all of this there was competition among agencies in presenting programs for the middle class for the young adults and for the better educated. But in the sixties the new concern to reach the undereducated gained momentum and in more than any other way the nature of agency programs changed to show this concern.

Resources

Adult educators have awakened to the resources now available to reach people in a more effective way in classrooms and in more creative ways outside of classrooms. Although the evidence from the Johnstone study in 1962 showed surprising little viewing of television for educational purposes, television is an accepted device at the disposal of the adult educators. The telephone, long neglected as a device for extending educational programs, has been creatively used by the Extension Service of the University of Wisconsin and a few other institutions. The developments of projection techniques in the audiovisual field have made no business or industry in-service program complete without the use of overhead projectors and similar machines to demonstrate processes, product, and progress. Adult educators have accepted the potential of modern technology and are creating new educational uses for it. Everything from the century-old telephone to the modern teaching machine and video tape recorder is part of the resource pool.

There has been a vast increase in funding for adult education. The federal government has been involved since the mid 1800s; some states since as early as the 1880s; local units of government from the mid 1700s; business, industries and professions since prehistory; and individuals as far back as history records. Yet it is only within this century that general commitments by federal, state, and local governments, by business, industry, and professions and by individuals have been made with such firmness that long term planning and organization can be developed with assurance that the resources to do the job are available.

THE FUTURE

Adult education is no longer on the margin of one's life in the United States. Adult and continuing education are part of the American way of life. This is as the early dreamers believed it should be. Recent changes in America suggest that adult education will have greater and greater impact. The three day weekends that are with us, the longer vacation periods that are being won in negotiations between union and management, the shorter working hours in some industries, the shorter work week in business and the earlier retirement all open more potentials for adult education. It may be natural for the human animal to adjust to his initial freedom from the long work week by a move to a total noninvolvement that can be gained from television or nonparticipant athletics. Yet this vegetarian response to leisure is ill-suited to intelligent beings for a long period. Adult educators should be prepared for the awakening of personal growth motives. They are beginning to appear. There are institutional bases upon which programs to meet personal growth motives can be built. The creative adult educator and his agency should be prepared to respond to the pressures for the positive use of nonwork time. The most appropriate and positive response could as likely come from the health professions as from agriculture; as likely from the electronics industry as from the unions; as likely from the universities as from the secondary schools. The impact of adult education on American society can be as great as the learners, the institutions, and the adult educators choose to make it.

Notes

1. Webster E. Cotton, *On Behalf of Adult Education*, Center for the Study of Liberal Education for Adults, Boston University, Brookline, Massachusetts, 1968.

2. A. A. Liveright, *A Study of Adult Education in the United States*, Center for the Study of Liberal Education for Adults at Boston University, 1968.

3. Webster E. Cotton, *On Behalf of Adult Education A Historical Examination of the Supporting Literature*, Center for the Study of Liberal Education for Adults at Boston University, 1968.

4. Knowles, Malcolm S., *The Adult Education Movement in the United States*, Holt, Rinehart and Winston, Inc., 1962.

5. Allen Tough, *The Adult's Learning Projects*, A Fresh Approach to Theory and Practice in Adult Learning, The Ontario Institute for Studies in Education, Toronto, Ontario, Canada, 1971.

REFERENCES

Axford, Roger W., *Adult Education: The Open Door*, International Textbook Co., Scranton, Pennsylvania, 1969.

Chiera, E., *They Wrote on Clay: The Babylonian Tablets Speak Today*, The University of Chicago Press, 1966.

Cotton, Webster E., *On Behalf of Adult Education: A Historical Examination of the Supporting Literature*, Center for the Study of Liberal Education for Adults at Boston University, Brookline, Massachusetts, 1968.

Grattan, C. H., *American Ideas about Adult Education (1710-1951)*, Bureau of Publications, Columbia University, New York, 1959.

Knowles, Malcolm S., *Handbook of Adult Education in the United States*, Adult Education Association, U.S.A., Washington, D.C., 1960.

Knowles, Malcolm S., *The Adult Education Movement in the United States*, Holt, Rinehart and Winston, Inc., New York, 1963.

Lindeman, Eduard C., *The Meaning of Adult Education*, Harvest House, Montreal, 1961.

Liveright, A. A., *A Study of Adult Education in the United States*, Center for the Study of Liberal Education for Adults at Boston University, Brookline, Massachusetts, 1968.

Roy, Nikhel R., *Adult Education in India and Abroad*, S. Chand and Co., Delhi, India, 1967.

Stobart, J. C., *The Glory that was Greece: A Survey of Hellenic Culture and Civilization*, Hawthorn Books, New York, 1964.

Styler, W. E., *Adult Education in India*, Oxford University Press, Apollo Bunder, Bombay 1, India, 1966.

Tough, Allen, *The Adult's Learning Projects: A Fresh Approach to Theory and Practice in Adult Learning*, The Ontario Institute for Studies in Education, Toronto, Ontario, Canada, 1971.

Wilson, John A., *The Burden of Egypt: An Introduction of Ancient Egyptian Culture*, The University of Chicago Press, 1951.

4

A philosophy of continuing education

There is an old and oft-repeated story about the university professor who vacationed one year in a remote Wisconsin village. He insisted upon being called "Dr. Jones," so one day the village grocer asked him, "What are you a doctor of?" The professor replied, "I'm a doctor of philosophy." The grocer scratched his head thoughtfully, and said, "I guess we don't have much of that around here."

To some extent nursing is like that Wisconsin village: we do not seem to have much philosophy. In the past, nurses have been primarily doers and not theorists, and if much thought were given to a philosophy of nursing, it was not recorded in the nursing literature. In recent years, however, several thoughtful and perceptive nurses have attempted to define their philosophies of nursing. In the emergence of nursing as a profession, these statements of philosophy are highly significant, particularly as they stimulate additional thought on the subject.

Although most readers will be familiar with these important writings, it may be useful to review them as one thinks about his own philosophy of continuing education. (See references at the end of the chapter.)

A viable philosophy of continuing education encompasses various aspects of life and is not limited to professional education. Thus continuing education is concerned with the development of the nurse as a person, a practitioner, and a citizen. These aspects of continuing education are often closely interrelated, but each must be considered in identifying a philosophy of education.

This chapter is designed to assist readers to think through their personal philosophies of continuing education. The content reflects the point of view of one of the authors and is presented as just that: one person's beliefs about continuing education. As with any philosophy of education, the authors recognize that there are differing points of view, and that there is no such thing as *the* philosophy of continuing education.

An individual's philosophy of continuing education in nursing is a reflection of many beliefs: his philosophy of life, of nursing, and of education. The nurse experienced in continuing education has identified his own philosophy of nursing, so this will be discussed only briefly in this chapter. As the educator thinks about his philosophy of education, it is important to keep his philosophy of nursing in mind. These two concepts seem quite compatible: most philosophies of nursing place an emphasis on the individual patient; current philosophies of continuing education focus on the individual learner.

WHAT IS PHILOSOPHY?

Philosophy may be literally translated as *love of wisdom* (from the Greek *philos*, meaning fond of, and *sophos*, meaning wise), but in its more usual connotation, philosophy is thought of as relating to basic beliefs. Actions are guided by one's beliefs; how one teaches relates to his beliefs about learning and about education.

Since philosophy provides a direction for action, it is useful to think through one's personal philosophy. It is possible that many persons do not think a great deal about their personal philosophy of life, yet what they do is based on the beliefs and values they hold.

To a great extent, the teacher's philosophy of education evolves from his philosophy of life. It is helpful, then, for the educator to think through his personal values and beliefs. For some, it may be useful to put these beliefs in writing; such an exercise may help the person determine those basic beliefs and values that serve as guideposts to personal action.

As with one's philosophy of life, one's personal philosophy of education is expressed not by what he says he believes, but by what he does. In the past, it was not uncommon for teachers to say they subscribed to a democratic philosophy, when in fact they taught in a very autocratic manner. What one believes about learning, the rights of the individual, and the needs of society are all reflected in one's approach to teaching. This is philosophy in action.

Philosophy is based on values deemed important, and the decisions one makes about content and methods of teaching are based on one's philosophy. In a period of rapid social changes, traditional values are questioned. Eternal truths no longer seem eternal. The thoughtful teacher recognizes that one's philosophy of education is always an emerging one, rather than a static one.

ELEMENTS OF CONTINUING EDUCATION

The practice of one's profession is only one part, albeit an important part, in the total life of any person. Therefore, if continuing education is to have meaning for each person, it must be broader than just that required to maintain professional competence.

To reiterate, philosophies of continuing education in nursing recognize the learner as a person, as a nurse, and as a citizen. The focus in the content of this book is largely limited to continuing education as it relates to nursing practice, but the importance of lifelong learning to personal growth and citizenship responsibilities is also recognized, and cannot be completely separated from continuing professional education. Thus continuing education is seen as a totality, and a sound philosophy of education recognizes all three aspects of lifelong learning.

This does not mean that the nurse educator is responsible for all three elements of continuing education. He is not equipped to take on such a responsibility but more than that, by offering nonnursing courses in the nursing department he may discourage nurses from participating in a wide range of educational pursuits. Diversity is part of the learning process and contributes to the development of the individual.

An example of a non nursing course that may be cited is music appreciation for nurses, which is sometimes offered by continuing education departments. One cannot deny the value of such courses to the personal development of the nurse, but one can question the appropriateness of the offering for the nursing department and the use of nursing time in the development of nonnursing courses. The only plausible argument is that nurses would not otherwise participate in them, which seems unlikely. These activities may tend to encourage provincialism among nurses, at a time when broader community involvement is needed. In most instances, however, the nurse benefits by learning with persons from other walks of life.

The nurse educator who accepts the concept of lifelong learning understands that he has a limited role in the development of the learner. But he also understands his responsibility to encourage nurses to recognize the value of participating in different types of educational activity. This requires that the educator be aware of sources of information about related continuing education activities.

THE INDIVIDUAL LEARNER

Any philosophy of continuing education recognizes each individual as a whole person. In his lifetime, each person plays many different roles. As an adult, the nurse may be a wife, mother, den mother, Sunday school teacher, a member of the PTA, nursing organization, and mental health association, and a citizen in the community in which she lives, to name some of these roles. Transcending all these roles, each person is an individual, with unique characteristics and personal interests. For every aspect of life, there are some continuing education elements.

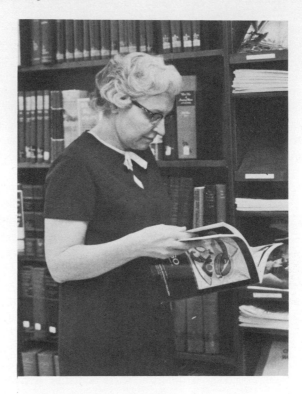

Figure 4-1 Individual library research is an important aspect of continuing professional education. (*Gary Schulz, University of Wisconsin Extension*)

Broadly speaking, the purpose of adult education is to help the individual become a more effective adult. Therefore, any philosophy of continuing education focuses on the individual learner, and is basic to the concept of self-directed learning. The right and the responsibility of the adult to direct his own learning is inherent in such a philosophy (Fig. 4-1).

Traditionally, most nurses have not been exposed to the concept of personal responsibility for their own continuing education. Such a concept may be seen as a requirement for survival in a society changing as rapidly as ours. Learning how to learn becomes a very significant aspect of such a concept.

Motivation

Motivation of the individual learner is a significant factor in the learning process, and some understanding of motivation is reflected in one's philosophy of continuing education. Motivation is a fascinating subject—ask any teacher who has observed a gifted student satisfied with getting by, or, conversely, a highly motivated, though less talented, student surpass the other members of his class. In spite of considerable research on the subject, much remains to be discovered about motivation.

How can nurses be motivated to accept personal responsibility for their own continued learning? There are no simple answers to the question, but a few ideas are worthy of consideration. Arousing the interest of the learner is one obvious motivating factor. Involving the learner in planning, designing activities that encourage participation, and stimulating new areas of interest are all significant.

It is apparent that internal motivation—the personal needs or desire to learn—is more effective than external incentives such as certificates, grades, credits, and the like. Since learning is closely related to need, many nurses will continue to seek learning opportunities as required by their work experience. Expanding opportunities for nurses, with emerging and changing roles, will increase these demands.

Specific continuing education requirements for licensure are external incentives, and for this reason are of questionable effectiveness as motivation for learning. A person may attend the prescribed number of class hours, and thus appear to meet the requirements, but if he is not interested in the content, and does not master it, the requirement is selfdefeating, for it may result in a distaste for further education.

The truly motivated person will learn without external requirements being placed upon him. He learns because he wants to learn, and because he has a need for the knowledge. As Dewey reminded us, the time to learn something is when you need to know it.

For the motivated learner, difficulties encountered in the process are seen as challenges, not as obstacles. A familiar example is the nurse who travels 100 miles to attend a conference which meets his learning needs; an unmotivated nurse will make no effort to attend, even if the conference is offered in his own community. Most of us know nurses who completed requirements for a college degree under very difficult circumstances: often while they were working, perhaps even full-time, carrying heavy family responsibilities, frequently traveling some distance. These were highly motivated nurses.

Involvement in the Learning Process

A philosophy of continuing education that places emphasis on the learner recognizes the importance of participation to the learning process. No matter how skillful teachers become at presenting content, nor how much visual aids are perfected, learning depends upon the student himself. A basic principle of education, often overlooked, is that *learning can be done only by the learner.*

The overuse or misuse of films, television, gimmicks, and so on, sometimes results in students confusing learning with entertainment. There is no magic road to learning, and though some ways of presenting content is more interesting or valuable than others, learning itself depends upon the effort put forth by the learner. This may be a difficult concept to grasp in a society where we demand so much instant action or instant answers to perplexing problems.

An appreciation of nurses as individuals is in sharp contrast to early educational patterns in nursing where attempts were made to mold students into standard behavior patterns. The unusual or different student was considered a maverick in nursing; often he was encouraged or even requested to leave the school. This traditional approach in schools of nursing no doubt accounts for some of the lack of leadership faced by the profession today. Nursing education has a long history of authoritarianism, a tradition that was further entrenched by rigid relationships with medical authority.

In addition to changing attitudes about students, an increased emphasis on lifelong learning by faculty in schools of nursing will change the expectation of tomorrow's nurse practitioner. Continuing education as a requirement for professional practice will be more generally accepted as a personal responsibility if faculty members serve as role models for continued educational pursuit.

Organized Learning Experiences

Placing the responsibility for learning on the learner does not preclude the need for formal continuing education programs. On the contrary, with rapidly expanding technical knowledge, and breathtaking social changes, it may mean just the reverse. But it does suggest that the learner be involved more directly in program planning and in the conduct of courses, as well as deciding which educational experiences are most suitable to him.

With the emphasis on the individual, organized learning activities are planned around the learner's needs. This suggests the importance of the learner's identification of his own needs, and his participation in determining appropriate learning activities. It further implies that those responsible for planning and conducting educational activities are able to assess the learning needs of participants. Finally, it suggests that the effective educator will have considerable understanding about learners as individuals.

A philosophy of continuing education recognizes the learner as an adult who accepts the responsibility for his own continuing learning. A belief in and respect for each person and an appreciation of individual differences are reflected in this philosophy. Translated into action, this means that these factors are recognized in program planning and design.

THE NEEDS OF SOCIETY

The aims of continuing education are broader than merely adding to the professional competence of the practitioner. When continued learning results in improved nursing practice, its social usefulness is obvious. Professional education also includes an increased understanding of the world in which one lives, so that the practitioner recognizes the importance of his contribution to the society of which he is a part and the significance of his work to the common good.

The perplexing problems of an increasingly complex society place more demands on citizens. Finding satisfactory solutions to these problems requires more knowledge and an increased understanding by all members of society. The need for education in these areas is apparent.

Many of the current problems of modern society bear a direct relationship to the health of the members of that society, and are of primary concern to all health professionals. Pollution in its various forms—air, water, noise—all have an adverse effect upon health. Overpopulation and increased urbanization multiply health problems in the affected areas. To a marked degree, these problems have a direct relationship to the concerns of nurses for the health of individuals, and nurses often have special contributions to make as solutions are sought. The extent of that contribution depends upon the interest of the nurse, his willingness to participate in community affairs, and his knowledge and understanding of the specific problem.

Quality of life is an overused expression that has almost become trite. Yet a concern for the quality of life is one mark of the educated person. It is not enough, for example, that modern medicine has extended the life expectancy; of equal concern is the kind of life the person is able to live in the society that has supported the research that results in a longer life span.

As the proportion of the population over age 65 increases, nurses must be increasingly aware of the needs of older people: economic, social, housing, recreation, health. Continuing education can contribute to meeting those needs in ways that are yet essentially untapped. Preretirement planning is an important aspect of continuing education; so is education designed specifically for what is euphemistically called the "golden years."

Modern technology has created a plethora of problems with moral, ethical, and legal overtones. The availability of heroic lifesaving measures has implications for the right of the individual to determine his own destiny. Transplantation of body organs has raised questions about the definition of death. Population pressures have resulted in new approaches to the issues of birth control and abortion.

The simplistic solutions to problems in a less complex and slower moving society are not adequate for today. The serious concerns of society demand innovative solutions, but also require approaches that are sound, reasonable, and humane. Such approaches will demand the best thinking available, and sound thinking on these urgent issues requires adequate information and a philosophical base.

In at least one university, a philosopher has been added to the faculty of the college of engineering. Perhaps colleges of nursing and medicine could emulate this idea; as technology advances, the human problems become more critical, and finding satisfactory solutions demands nontraditional approaches.

The critical issues facing society can only be met by a concerned, well-informed citizenry, who are willing to devote thought, time, and energy to their solution. In a truly democratic society, the citizens are vitally concerned and actively involved in seeking solutions to the problems faced by that society. Adequate preparation for participatory democracy is probably the most important contribution of continuing education.

Universal education of children is sometimes identified as the most significant American contribution of the nineteenth century. Perhaps universal continuing education will become a reality before the close of the present century. Though not uniquely American, this contribution could be of comparable significance.

The New Leisure

An increase in the amount of leisure time available to larger numbers of people has implications for both the individual and society. There is concern that unless individuals learn how to use leisure time constructively, that time will be used for destructive purposes. Therefore, the wise use of leisure time is an urgent need for society, and one to which continuing education should address itself.

Increased mechanization has led to a shorter work week for many industrial workers, and eventually this change, along with a different time organization for the work week, will affect nursing practice. The shorter work week will also have an impact upon nurses themselves, since it will result in increased leisure. The availability of time will permit the nurse to participate in more educational activities; whether he will, in fact, use the time for this purpose is yet to be determined. Unless he gives it a high priority, his leisure time will not be used for educational purposes.

Planning for increased leisure time is appropriate for nurses, as well as for members of other occupational groups. Will nurses use the new leisure in constructive ways—or will a lack of thought and preparation result in boredom and frustration and other nonconstructive uses of increasing amounts of available time? Continuing education could help provide the answer to this question.

CONTINUING PROFESSIONAL EDUCATION

The focus of this book is on continuing education for the professional nurse, a major concern for the serious practitioner. The plea of the authors is that nurse educators recognize continuing professional education as only one facet of lifelong learning, and place it in its proper perspective.

Philosophy of Nursing

The educator's philosophy of continuing nursing education rests with his basic beliefs about nursing practice. If he sees nursing with a primary emphasis on concern for the individual patient, his teaching will be directed to those concerns. Conversely, if he believes that nursing is primarily task-oriented, his approach will be quite different.

Developing a sound philosophy of nursing may not be easy, whether for the individual practitioner or for the nursing profession as such. Can nursing have a philosophy apart from medicine? Perhaps some of the conflicts between nurses and physicians are the result of divergent operational philosophies of care. If nurses accept their role as primarily that of the patient advocate, the breach between medical and nursing practice may widen.

In developing a philosophy of nursing, the kind of society in which we live must be considered. Nursing is based on a concept of service, and this is difficult to reconcile in a society which appears to be based on a materialistic philosophy. (Each year, for example, in this country we spend more federal funds on highways than on higher education).

The educator's philosophy of nursing colors his view of the practitioner. If he sees nurses as professional persons, he respects their independence and autonomy. He expects them to be self-directed learners, and he encourages them in their efforts. In program planning, he does not avoid controversial content, but is aware that conflicting points of view are valuable to the learning process.

The educator whose philosophy of nursing encompasses a concern for the individual patient will have no difficulty accepting a philosophy of continuing education that emphasizes the individual learner. The great divergency in preparatory nursing programs presents a challenge to the continuing education faculty. Accepting the individual learner means acknowledging these divergent backgrounds.

A concern for the individual learner requires understanding and compassion by the faculty member. But above all, it requires the skill to help the person recognize his own potential and make the most of it. The German poet Goethe said it best: "If we take people as they are, we make them worse. If we treat them as if they were what they ought to be, we help them become what they are capable of becoming."

Liberal Education and Nursing

Certain aspects of liberal education may be seen as an integral part of nursing education; other aspects may not be directly related. Sometimes it is difficult to separate the two: if the nurse is learning Spanish to prepare himself to work as a nurse with the Peace Corps in Peru, the two aspects are very closely related.

Historically, education for professionals encompassed considerable liberal education, so the practitioners in the traditional professions (law, medicine, and theology) were educated in the broad sense of the term. The rapid expansion of knowledge necessary to the effective practice of medicine has forced medical schools to increase technical content in curriculums with an accompanying reduction in liberal studies. This is paradoxical at a time when the ethical and moral issues relating to medical practice are becoming increasingly more complex, and physicians (and others) must have a sound and broad basis on which to make wise decisions. One would not wish for a return of the horse and buggy doctor, but one might hope for more physicians with the broad knowledge and understanding of a Dr. Osler.

Continuing education for the physician, as for other professionals, tends to be limited to technical content. For the most part, adult education has provided opportunities for practitioners to improve their occupational (and economic) status, but has generally failed to provide that education which would contribute to a better understanding of the world in which they live. One cannot blame the educational institutions alone for this failure. For the most part, institutions respond to needs, and this need has not been identified by practitioners. Realistically, it is also recognized that the demand for keeping up with professional study alone is almost overwhelming.

As colleagues, nurses are concerned with physicians' loss of status and prestige. Although this change is assuredly not the result of only one factor, one might speculate if the patients' loss of trust is not, in part, related to the decreased amount of liberal studies in the education of today's physician. He is forced to become a technician at a time when the world needs more humanitarians, a role he is no longer prepared to assume.

This change in the education of physicians is of major concern to nurses. In some instances, it means that the nurse may have a broader understanding of the complex social issues than the physician.

The proportion of liberal education in most nursing curriculums has increased steadily over the past twenty years. Yet it is obvious that future practice will place heavy demands on all the health professionals, and that effective, humane practice requires practitioners with the insight, understanding, and attitudes that are difficult to teach in professionally oriented courses.

Why liberal education for nurses? Perhaps this story relating to adult education in Denmark best illustrates the reason. A Danish farmer went to enroll his son in one of the folk schools of Bishop Grundtvig, the founder of the Danish adult education movement. The folk schools were nonvocational, but the farmer inquired if his son would learn how to make better butter. "No," said Grundtvig, "We will not teach him how to make better butter." "Then," said the farmer, "what will he learn?" "My friend," was Grundtvig's reply, "If your boy graduates from the folk school, for the rest of his life he will be ashamed to make inferior butter."

If it achieves its goal, continuing education will make the nurse ashamed to give less than quality care to patients. Continuing liberal education becomes an imperative for professional practice.

Interprofessional Continuing Education

Interdisciplinary approaches to continuing education for health professionals appears to be an imperative for the future. It seems logical that those who work together learn together, and in fact, some preparatory educational programs now include course content open to all those in various health fields. With this education background, perhaps it can be assumed that the future graduates of these programs will not only expect more interdisciplinary continuing education, but will be more ready to accept it. Present practitioners may not be easily convinced, but some efforts are being directed to interdisciplinary educational approaches.

Even if one accepts wholeheartedly the concept of interprofessional continuing education, the educator must recognize that such programming is rather complex. An effective interdisciplinary course requires input from all professional groups for whom it is intended. In the past, too many so-called interdisciplinary courses have been designed by members of one discipline for other health professionals. Decisions about content of such programs were made arbitrarily by those offering them on the basis of content they deemed necessary for participants, without any involvement of the latter. If a program is to be truly interdisciplinary, all the appropriate groups must be involved from the outset.

In the immediate future, interdisciplinary education may be largely an adjunct to, and not a replacement for, educational activities designed for those in a specific field. Nevertheless, the benefits of planning and learning together are considerable, and present efforts in this direction are encouraging.

THE ROLE OF EDUCATIONAL INSTITUTIONS

Expanding needs and desires for continuing education will place increasing demands on all educational institutions. Tax-supported institutions have a particular responsibility for providing educational opportunities for adult learners, but in the future the entire load of continuing education cannot be carried by the universities. However, they will undoubtedly be expected to assume the greater share of the responsibility.

With an increasing number of agencies involved in continuing education, coordination becomes more complex. Without coordination, efforts are duplicated and resources wasted, and educational gaps occur. A clear understanding of responsibilities is required to use existing resources to good advantage. For example, a university should not offer sessions that are more suitable as hospital in-service programs; the reverse is also true.

In addition to providing increasing opportunities for continuing education, the university has a responsibility for educating the adult educator. Priorities may need to be established in terms of educational spin-off, to use the parlance of the day. This refers to multiplying the effect of educating one person who in turn educates others. Thus, in nursing, the university may have a special responsibility for preparing the nurse educators in in-service departments, for these persons teach many different employees who benefit indirectly from the original teaching.

The professions have long held a recognized place within the university for the education of practitioners. For the emerging professions, such as nursing, that place is somewhat more tenuous and of more recent origin. Thus, the institution may be slow to accept its role in continuing nursing education as well as in the preparatory or advanced programs.

The Preparatory Program and Continuing Education

Emerson reminds us that "the things taught in colleges and schools are not an education, but the means to an education." Schools of nursing are beginning to accept their responsibility not only for teaching students the need for lifelong learning for professional practice but also for helping them identify and locate appropriate learning resources for continued study. Helping the individual learn how to learn is another important function of preparatory nursing programs.

Unfortunately, students in nursing do not see many nurses who are continuing learners. For too long nurses finished their educations when they were graduated from the school of nursing; even today it is not unusual to hear a nurse brag that he has not "cracked a book" since he left school. Demands required by rapid changes have stimulated learning in many instances, but traditions are not altered overnight.

Some faculty members have always been continuing learners, but even among this group those learners were probably exceptional. The writer recalls the surprised student she met in the library, who exclaimed, "What are *you* doing in the library?" the implication being that faculty are not usually found in the library.

Modern approaches to nursing education encourages thoughtful questioning of existing practices. Such questioning is desperately needed in nursing, but this approach must be based on sound knowledge and careful analysis. This implies continued study by the questioner.

The Teacher in Continuing Education

The role of the teacher in continuing education is discussed in Chapter 7, but a consideration of this role as it relates to philosophy may be helpful, since the teacher's approach is based on his own beliefs about learning. Effective adult educators support the concept of self-directed learning.

We do nurses a disservice by making them too dependent upon the teacher, and it is easy to do this, for this is the type of education most familiar to the nurse. Too often dependency results from the teacher's own needs: the dependence of the learner helps the teacher feel important. Dependence is encouraged by teachers who plan content down to the last minute and including every detail, who always provide answers to the students' questions, who discourage self-discovery.

With a recognition of the independence of the adult learner, the teacher's role becomes an assistive rather than a prescriptive one. He helps the learner diagnose his own learning needs, plan for his own educational activities, and discover how to locate and use educational resources. As Rheba de Tornyay has pointed out, "the function of higher education is not teaching—it is bringing about learning."[1] This is particularly true in continuing education.

In continuing education, self-direction is an important aspect of planning. Involvement and participation are essential, with a recognition that both may take various forms. For example, an inspiring lecture can motivate the learner, but a packed program of lectures, no matter how good, can result in boredom and loss of interest without the opportunity for thought or exchange of ideas. Encouraging nurses to build on their present knowledge and to seek additional sources of information requires special skill.

In the past the teacher was seen as a dispenser of knowledge, and the learner as a passive recipient. With the rapid advancement of knowledge today, many adult learners may know more than the teacher about some things.

When learners are recognized as colleagues, and when it is accepted that students and teachers are learning together, the role of the teacher becomes different from the traditional one. The teacher's aim must be to assist learners to become capable, independent thinkers with considerable judgment, decision-making skill, and problem-solving ability. His actions are supported by his philosophy of learning.

Notes

1. Rheba de Tornyay, *Strategies for Teaching Nursing*, John Wiley and Sons, Inc., New York, 1971, p. 132.

REFERENCES

American Nurses' Association: *Avenues for Continued Learning*, The Association, New York, 1967.

Augenstein, Leroy G.: *Come, Let Us Play God*, Harper and Row, New York, 1969.

Bradford, Leland: "Toward a Philosophy of Adult Education," *Adult Education*, 7(2): 83-93, 1957.

Brunner, Edmund DeS.: *An Overview of Adult Education Research*, Adult Education Association, Chicago, 1959.

Bryson, Lyman: *Adult Education*, American Book Company, New York, 1936.

Bullough, Bonnie, and Vern Bullough (eds.): *New Directions for Nurses*, Springer Publishing Company, New York, 1971.

Cooper, Signe S.: "Continuing Education: An Imperative for Nursing," *Nurs. Forum*, 7(3): 289-297, 1968.

Dorland, James R.: "Current Issues in Adult Education," *Adult Lead.*, 15(10): 349-350; 381-383, 1967.

Elkins, Wilson H.: "Education is Continuous," *Nurs. Outlook*, 9(4): 243-245, 1961.

Fisher, Dorothy Canfield: *Why Stop Learning?* Harcourt, Brace and Company, New York, 1927.

Gnagey, Theodore: "The Coming Revolution in Education," *Adult Education*, 15(1): 9-16, 1964.

Henderson, Virginia: *The Nature of Nursing*, The Macmillan Company, New York, 1966.

Johnson, Dorothy: "The Significance of Nursing Care," *Amer. J. Nurs.*, 61(11): 63-66, 1961.

Kallen, Horace M.: "On Liberating Adults: A Philosophy for Adult Educators," *Adult Lead.*, 13(4): 98-100; 119-121, 1964.

Kidd, J. R.: *How Adults Learn*, Association Press, New York, 1960.

Kilpatrick, William Heard: "The Task Confronting Adult Education," *J. of Adult Educ.*, 1(4): 403-412, 1929.

Knowles, Malcolm D.: "Philosophical Issues That Confront Adult Education," *Adult Education*, 7(4): 234-240, 1957.

————: *The Modern Practice of Adult Education*, Association Press, New York, 1970.

Kuehn, Ruth Perkins: "Continuing Education in Nursing," *J. Amer. Med. Assn.*, 190(6): 544-545, 1964.

Lindeman, Eduard C.: *The Meaning of Adult Education*, New Republic, Inc., New York, 1926.

Morton, John R.: *University Extension in the United States*, University of Alabama Press, Birmingham, 1953.

Nahm, Helen: "Changing Attitudes and Approaches to Nursing Care Through Continuing Education," *J. Nurs. Educ.*, 8(3): 31-36, 1969.

Nightingale, Florence: *Notes on Nursing: What It Is, and What It Is Not*, facsimile of the 1st ed., London, 1859, J. B. Lippincott, Philadelphia, 1946.

Ohliger, John, and Colleen McCarthy: *Lifelong Learning or Lifelong Schooling? A Tentative View of the Ideas of Ivan Illich with A Quotational Bibliography*, Publications in Continuing Education, Syracuse University and ERIC Clearinghouse on Adult Education, Syracuse, New York, 1971.

Olson, Edith: "Education for—What?" *Amer. J. Nurs.*, 70(7): 1508-1510, 1970.

Osler, Sir William: *Aequanimitas and other Papers That Have Stood the Test of Time*, W. W. Norton and Company, Inc., New York, 1963.

Powell, John Walker: *Learning Comes of Age*, Association Press, New York, 1956.

Reiter, Frances: "The Nurse-Clinician," *Amer. J. Nurs.*, 66(2): 274-280, 1966.

Shannon, Theodore J., and Clarence A. Schoenfeld: *University Extension*, The Center for Applied Research in Education, New York, 1965.

Sheats, Paul H.: "New Knowledge for What?" *Adult Lead.*, 11(7): 194-196; 221-222, 1963.

Thorndike, Edward L., et al.: *Adult Learning*, The Macmillan Company, New York, 1928.

Toffler, Alvin: *Future Shock*, Random House, Inc., New York, 1970.

Verner, Coolie, with the assistance of Alan Booth: *Adult Education*, The Center for Applied Research in Education, Inc., New York, 1964.

Wiedenback, Ernestine: *Clinical Nursing: A Helping Art*, Springer Publishing Company, New York, 1964.

5

Principles of
adult education

Because continuing nursing education is seen as a part of the adult education effort in general, guidelines which are emerging in that field are relevant to nursing. Previous chapters provided a broad base for understanding the place of continuing nursing education in society today. The need to develop and expand the efforts in this aspect of professional education was emphasized, and historical roots for programming were traced. Trends in adult education were reviewed and some important beliefs about continuing education were considered. In logical sequence then, extension of some ideas alluded to earlier is now appropriate.

In adapting from the adult education field to nursing education, a commonality is readily identifiable in the term *education*. Recognition of education as an applied science is important. Knowledge derived from the biological, behavioral, and social sciences forms the foundations for principles of adult education. As that knowledge is used and applied to the teaching-learning process, it takes on added zest and meaning when personally experienced.

Nurses have long been familiar with phrases such as the principles of nursing or the principles of patient care. So, words like *the principles of adult education* may arouse positive feelings of approval and anticipation of some practical guidelines. However, broad principles applied to a specific situation may require careful interpretation. Recognizing that adaptations or modifications of principles are a possibility, a review of principles may be helpful. A principle is defined here to mean an element or quality which produces a specific effect. The effect specified and desired is learning.

EXTENDING LEARNING

In the mid-1960s, a publication written by Burton W. Kreitlow reported a project endorsed by the Commission of Professors, Adult Education Association

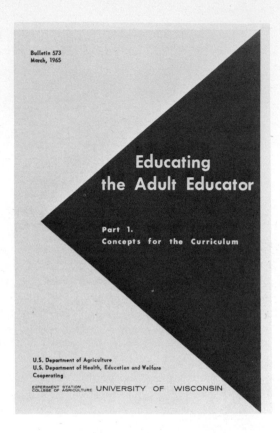

Figure 5-1   Educating the adult educator.

of the U.S.A.[1] Kreitlow found that, prior to 1961, published research literature related to the education of adults was sparse. As an adult educator of student adult educators, his concern was to search out relevant research (Fig. 5-1). He noted that the fields of cooperative extension, psychology, sociology, anthropology, vocational education, industrial relations, social welfare, executive training, and communications were among those adding to useful research reports.

In addition to Kreitlow, several other authors have contributed to the work of summarizing pertinent research. References to these contributions are found at the end of this chapter. Although some studies appear to be far removed from nursing, they may have a direct impact on nursing. For example, agricultural research on the process of innovation, diffusion, and adoption of farm practices is of interest to both nursing service and nursing education. In the former, a replication study in the areas of the team concept, nursing audit, or unit dose system of medication administration would be interesting. In the latter, studies in adoption of curriculum approaches, methods of teaching, or evaluation of learning would be exciting. Although the practices differ between farming and nursing, is the process of innovation, diffusion, and adoption as identified by agricultural research basically the same?

In another area of research, the constraints that have inhibited the broad adult education efforts may easily be translated to nursing. The constraints from some adult learning theories have their origin in certain early studies. Generalizations and interpretations drawn from studies which may be historic but do not apply to today's world are of questionable validity regarding modern adults. For example, Kidd reviews and discusses evidence from various studies based on the use of intelligence tests.[2] He points out that in one study at time of testing, the younger members of the test group had much more formal schooling than the older members, a fact which was considered irrelevant then but is not so considered today. Another limiting factor of early studies such as those conducted by E. L. Thorndike is related to age. The age range found in early test groups represented a time when the life span was much less than the present seventy years. More recent studies have included older people as subjects and have focused on learning ability. Earlier studies centered on the rate or speed of learning, sometimes described as learning efficiency.

The late Irving Lorge worked with the notion that perhaps there was more to learning than performance measured by getting certain tasks done in a given unit of time. Thus Lorge differentiated between learning performance and learning ability. He concluded that learning performance was affected by a variety of factors such as personal interests or reaction time due to deficits from the normal aging process. On the other hand, he equated learning ability with the power to learn. The outcomes from his studies provide clear evidence that between the ages of 20 and 60 years, significant changes in learning ability do not occur and that the 60-year-old maintains his power to learn.[3] Performance may decline but intelligence or learning ability does not.

Why, then, do adults tend to learn less than they might? Or to paraphrase the same question, why do nurses tend to learn less than they might? What are some reasons for the failure of nurses, particularly among older staff nurses, to become continuing learners in nursing?

FACTORS AND CONCEPTS IN LEARNING

In a youth-oriented culture, the fact of aging is borne because no choice exists. Youth has the image of vitality and action; aging, the image of limitations and inactivity. Youth is seen as the time for learning; age, as the time when it is too late to learn. Youth looks forward; age, backward. Such perceptions of differences that ages make have become ingrained in a youth-oriented culture and provided a disservice to all who share the distorted views. Therein may lie at least a partial explanation for the so-called generation gap.

Age and Feelings

Paradoxically, the older person may claim to have learned much from living and his experiences and at the same time say that he is too old to learn. The implication is that unplanned, incidental learning is acceptable; planned learning, formal or informal, is not. One unknown sage has pointed out that one reason experience is such a good teacher is that she does not allow any dropouts.

Reasons for rejecting planned learning may vary among older staff nurses as with any other group. People tend to be creatures of habit and habits are not easily broken. When learning habits are not a part of daily routine, conscious effort for a change is demanded. Routines also involve a time factor and a preestablished set of priorities. Is the individual willing or able to reorder his time and priorities? To what extent will the significant others in his life encourage or deter him from continuing education?

Sometimes guilt, fear, or lack of self-confidence are feelings which the older staff nurse may need to overcome before committing himself to a course of study. Time spent away from ward, spouse, family, housework, or social obligations for a personal, albeit professional, pursuit of learning may arouse guilt feelings in some nurses. Fear of failing to meet self-set expectations or those expectations he imagines others set for him may be sufficient deterrents to keep the nurse from joining a class. The lack of self-confidence may be because of an unfounded belief in limited learning capabilities. Brunner and his coresearchers have documented studies which support the belief that adults do learn less than they might.[4] Reasons cited include self-imposed limitations as a result of narrowing interests, and related attitudes and values held. Even adults under age 40 were found to lack confidence in personal ability to extend themselves beyond familiar or routine things.

Brunner and his colleagues also noted that highly anxious persons did not learn as rapidly as others in test situations.[5] Nurses are especially aware of the multiple causes of anxiety in patients yet may fail to recognize or accept their own anxieties as learners. In turn, the learner's anxiety level may be heightened if it is not recognized by the teacher. If to the anxiety is added the burden of long unused powers of learning, the reluctance to start learning experiences is understandable among, for example, some older staff nurses.

Yet, the adult can learn to learn. The adult's ability to learn is no longer questioned by psychologists and educational psychologists. However, the extent to which the adult may bestir himself to engage in learning activities may well depend on his desires or motivations.

Motivation

In the context of this chapter, the term *motivation* is equated with the desire to learn or interest in learning. While social psychologists explore the basic origins of motives, the educator confronting the continuing learner in nursing is faced with the result and reality of motivated behavior. Whether the action of the learner in being present for a learning experience is due to a basic instinct, innate drives, or goal-directed behavior, some incentive apparently prevailed. The concern of the teacher is then to determine which incentives they were and how they might affect learning, and to be aware of the effects of other motives on learning.

Lorge noted that although interest changes occurred with rapidity between 15 to 25 years of age, the interests of the 25-year-old were stable enough to serve as an indicator of his interests at a much later date.[6] Major shifts of interest may be attributed to either physical changes (sensory, motor, or other deficits) or social changes (new family responsibilities).

Just as the adult learner is capable of learning to learn, he is likewise capable of learning to become interested or motivated. Without a recognition of such capability, the teacher of adults may fall into the trap of programming solely on the basis of the learner's interests as expressed by them. Everyone will not follow the same pattern in developing interests nor will they all start or end with a common degree of motivation. Despite such variations, the teacher who is cognizant of student potentials will try to identify critical factors affecting motivation and incorporate into the teaching-learning process different ways of activating theory into practice. The next question may well be "What are some of the theoretical concepts?" A number of notions held by the experienced instructor who is interested in this aspect of learning have previously been validated by others through study of isolated incentives affecting motivation.[7] Repeated testings have shown that when the learner knows that he is to be provided with feedback on the work he does, his work goes up in quantity and accuracy, and involves less time. Conversely, if the student does not know the purpose of learning given tasks, not only does efficiency decrease but also the fatigue factor increases. Likewise, if the learner knows or feels a task is impossible to do, accomplishment decreases. Both a mild emotional tension and a reasonable limit on time, have a positive effect on accurate learning but too little or too much of either serve as constraints or interference to learning.

The foregoing concepts sound neither earth-shaking nor profound. Indeed, like many good continuing learners, we may have learned them from experience and derived the same conclusions on an intuitive basis. But scientific approval lends comfort and more. The translation into action is imperative.

To what extent do current programs provide feedback on learning tasks? Are the goals for educational programs carefully and practically developed for and with the adult learner rather than imposed as a set of grand and glorious teaching aims? For example, when the nurse instructor has the goal of providing learning experiences to enhance the teaching of patients but has not considered at all the circumstances in which students will be applying that learning, the teacher's goal may be unrealistic and irrelevant from the learner's point of view. Is thought given to the feasibility of a learning task and is it one which may be possible or impossible to accomplish without any interceding content or set of circumstances? Have the external or environmental and inter- and intrapersonal factors been considered to promote learning? Is the timing right, sufficient, and adequate? These are but a few questions which need answering before putting theory into practice.

The learners' self-expectations may influence and be influenced by their own past learning experiences. Thus, the saying "Nothing succeeds like success" is relevant to the teaching-learning process. The less successful perhaps believe that failure begets failure. At any rate, there is a social psychological concept of *level of aspiration* which relates to a sense of self and pride which the individual feels must be maintained. Experiments dealing with this concept have indicated that without previous experience on a given task, levels of aspiration were low; with experience, levels were changed and the direction of change was according to work as individuals rather than as a group. In relating the findings of studies on levels of aspiration to nursing, one may speculate that those individuals who feel the greatest personal need for the career ladder to progress from nursing assistant to practical nurse to technical nurse to professional nurse may be those whose levels and directions changed according to their own accomplishments. The student's self-expectations may not be consistent with the real world but because they are consistent with the learner's self-image, they affect motivation and must be taken into account. The continuum extends from a new graduate nurse who finished yesterday and may feel he knows what is important for today and tomorrow, to the older nurse who has worked for the last forty years and feels driven to keep up with the changing times.

Although external (behavioral) indicators of motivation are being sought, further research is needed before conclusive statements can be made. Factors such as persistence in attendance, distance traveled to a course, and choice of enrollment for particular courses may be indicators but are open to question when related to motivation. Unknown variables are suspected of introducing bias or clouding the clarity of behavior assigned to motives. Further, delineation of the underlying stimulus that initiated action toward adult education participation would be helpful.

R. G. Kuhlen spearheaded a systematic look at adult motivation and concluded that as the adult developed through the years and met varying life experiences at least two different kinds of motives were identifiable.[8] Kuhlen cites growth-expansion motives as dominant during the first half of adult life, with the effort to meet the needs engendered by the assuming of new responsibilities of adulthood, employment, marriage, family, and social life. As the years pass and individuals face the realities of grown children leaving home, retirement, and loss of spouse, anxiety or threat motives become dominant. Small wonder then that rigidity is sometimes equated with age. When an individual is threatened or anxious, he will use and cling to tried and tested ways of reducing such emotions from his own previous experiences. Rather than applying a label of rigidity, the adult educator is concerned about understanding the concept of set.

Set

The term *set* is a common enough word. In education, the teacher hopes the student has developed a learning set. In talking about certain individuals, the speaker may describe them as being set in their ways. The concept of set is generally recognized but may not be fully appreciated as an important consideration for the teaching-learning process.

If learning hinges on response, either covert or overt, set may be defined as a response that the particular individual has learned. Whether the individual learned the response through repetition and formed a habit or persisted in taking the line of least resistance is relatively immaterial. The important thing is that given a circumstance which the individual perceives as similar to those previously experienced, he will respond in a way which meets his needs.

Although the power to learn remains undiminished with advancing years, the rate or speed of learning slows. Add the habitual response or set to the decrease in speed of learning and the outcome may be a resistance to learning new responses. Learning different responses requires attention, effort, and involvement and may be viewed as just too much trouble.

Because a response is habitual does not necessarily mean that the set was derived without thought. On the contrary, some sets are solidly based on knowledge and understanding. In such instances, sets will serve either as an advantage or disadvantage to the individual involved, depending on the way he uses them. When sets are used constructively as points of departure for further learning, they are an advantage. If sets are used to dig in for a holding action to preclude or forestall new or different ideas, they are a distinct disadvantage. The adult's perception of time, schedules, and priorities may be a kind of set and in turn influence other sets.

The mix of mind and emotion present in a set is taken into account when working with the adult learner. A readiness to learn may not just happen. More often than not, whatever set is present requires recognition and respect while the teacher also focuses on assisting the learner to develop, through a step-by-step process, a readiness to learn. McClusky suggests that a program could well be designed in terms of the preparation, cumulation, and dissolution of sets, and the impact of these processes on goal achievement.[9] A nursing program using such an approach would be interesting indeed. Implications are inherent for nursing practice goals and for patient-teaching goals. For example, a program focusing on social problems affecting health and health care—such as the problem of alcoholism, where sets may involve mind, morality, and emotions—might lend itself to McClusky's suggested approach.

Differentiation

Nurses believe in the individuality and uniqueness of each patient so the concept of differentiation is not new to them, although the term may be unfamiliar. However, a discussion examining some of the concept's ramifications, as they relate to the teaching-learning process, may be useful.

Differentiation is possible and observable only because of identifiable, specific factors which account for the individuality of any person. Preferences, interests, abilities, and degrees of discrimination in particular situations are examples of factors from which specificity may be derived. Age, sex, level of schooling, and occupation are some other factors. While the list of examples is far from complete, a sense of personal orientation may be inferred. The individual or personal component of the concept of differentiation is readily recognized. Perhaps the social component is not as easily recognized.

The changes in social roles required during the life span force any person to engage in a variety of social interactions. A person forms relationships with others who may be changing even as he himself is changing. Personal, professional, and civic responsibilities demand more social expansion of the adult than of the child or youth. Obviously, individual responses to experiences vary just as the experiences themselves vary; and so it seems that the more experiences one has, the greater will be the range of differentiation from another with fewer experiences. Thus, if age bears a direct relationship to numbers of experiences, adults have a greater range of differentiation than children.

In working with the nurse learner, the instructor may wish to consider the following statements growing out of the concept of differentiation:

1. Adults are highly differentiated persons.
2. Adults' learning interests are specific to the individual.

Principles which may be derived from the foregoing statements are:

1. Design learning experiences to meet the particular needs of a selected group.
2. Organize learning experiences to evoke and expand specific interests of individuals.

Interesting though a program may be, the learning results will vary.
Humans are not always consistent beings and their learning performance is often
affected by internal factors or external pressures impinging on them. Sometimes
a great deal of learning occurs despite interference; sometimes the learning is
minimal through no fault of the curriculum. Seldom are one individual's efforts
maintained on a level plane over time. The uneven performance may be attributed to the load the person is carrying at a given time according to another adult
education concept which deals with margin.

Margin of Power

A fairly recent addition to the conceptual framework of the dynamics of
adult development and learning was to introduce by McClusky's approach to a
concept of *margin*.[10] In defining margin, McClusky used the words *load* and
power.

Load refers to the demands made on an individual by himself and society
and is divisible into two interacting elements, external load and internal load.[11]
External load consists of tasks in daily life involving—for example—relatives,
occupational, social, and civic obligations. Internal load consists of aspirations
and expectations set by the person for himself, such as the need to succeed or
the desire to excel.

Power as used by McClusky denotes the resources which the individual
draws upon to cope with his load. Power consists of multiple factors, such as
intellectual, social, physical, and economic abilities, which interact with one
another and with other learned skills to assist in the coping process for meeting
as effectively as possible the tasks of living.

Margin, then, is described as surplus power when power is greater than
load. However if the ratio of load to power is nearly 1.00, there may be very
surplus power, and margin is seen as a function of the relationship between the
designations in the ratio. To assure a margin of power, load will need to be
decreased or power increased. Provided the individual is not locked into a
circumstance which offers him no choices, some control of margin is possible.

But, with few or no choices, neither load nor power may be manipulated to obtain a greater margin of power.

In relating the concept of margin to the field of continuing education in nursing, familiar phrases come to mind such as, "I've had it! It's more than I can bear. I'm at my wit's end. If only I could get out from under." Such phrases suggest that a point of tolerance has been reached and the ratio of load to power leaves little margin for life's tasks. Add the task of continuing education to a nurse with that little margin and little, if any, learning is likely. Some adjustment in either load or power is indicated. But what are the choices? Is it possible to change the staffing pattern, use auxiliary personnel such as ward clerks, or initiate a new delivery system of medications and supplies to reduce the load? Is it possible to reorder priorities, reallocate time, or revise an approach to patient care to increase the power? If no choice exists, little change in margin is likely.

Conversely, with choices for autonomy or control, the margin is amenable to change. For example, let us say that some administrative changes are rumored, and the nurses who are likely to be affected are carrying a load of uncertainty. The future is not clear regarding individual placement on the kind of clinical unit, hours, position, or salary. When the guidelines for change are clarified and choices or options for those nurses are made known, the load may decrease. Thus, the margin may be increased because the surplus power is now increased.

Another way to increase power is to add to the number of the learned skills which help the nurse to cope more effectively with the load being faced. Time and motion studies in the work-simplification approach and continuing education in nursing supervision courses are examples of efforts to increase power and thereby increase the margin of power.

Changes in the load and power alluded to thus far have dealt with examples from the clinical life of the nurse. Yet margin is needed to meet other tasks of life as well, such as coping with changes in life roles.

Changes in Life Roles

Maslow relates basic needs or values to a growth and self-actualization psychology.[12] He describes a developmental system which is arranged in a hierarchical manner starting from purely biological or physiological needs, for example, food, fluids, shelter, and safety, and moving to the highest psychological need, which Maslow terms *general self-actualization*.[13] Only when the urgent life-preserving needs are adequately met, does Maslow's theory allow for fulfilling the next steps toward love or affection, then esteem or recognition needs. The continuum is seen as a being-and-becoming concept in which the dependency of immaturity is gradually replaced by responsible maturity which makes possible less self-consciousness, less selfishness, and more transcendence of self.[14]

In a very practical sense, Maslow's theory has many implications for continuing education in nursing. Starting with the physiological needs, the ubiquitous coffee break and meals become important. The classroom setting, ventilation, and seating arrangement may inhibit or foster learning conditions. Recognition of the individual learner as a person valued for himself may contribute to meeting his needs for affection and esteem, thus freeing him to devote the energy conserved from the struggle for esteem to learning for self-actualization.

Another fairly recent theory relating to changing roles and responsibilities in adult life was identified by Havighurst.[15] His theory includes two approaches to systematize adult development.

The first way Havighurst suggests is to view segments of adult life according to the developmental tasks required during any particular phase. Failure to achieve those tasks during the particular phase indicates a lack of competence for meeting future developmental tasks and makes success at future tasks less likely. Thus, when a particular task presents itself for learning within a certain time period, such as becoming a grandparent or entering retirement, these times are described as teachable moments.

The second way of approaching adult development, according to Havighurst, is to view the totality of adulthood as a set of changing social roles. He identifies such roles as worker, parent, spouse, and citizen and suggests they be subdivided according to young, middle, and older adults for educational program planning to help individuals improve performance in their roles.

Havighurst believes in two basic aspects of education, the instrumental and the expressive. Both are seen as essential for lifelong learning. He defines instrumental education as education for a goal which is external to the act of education. For example, the continuing learner in nursing may study electrocardiography to enable her to practice as a nurse in a coronary care unit. Education is the instrument by which the learner changes his situation. In return for an investment of time and energy, future gain is expected in instrumental education. In expressive education as explained by Havighurst, the education is for a goal which is so closely related to the act of learning that the act itself seems to be the goal. An example is the nurse who studies current nursing concepts for immediate application and because she enjoys learning more about the nursing process. Expressive education implies a present gain in return for the time and energy used. Both the instrumental and expressive aspects of education lend themselves to Havighurst's approaches to adulthood, whether it be the developmental task or social roles approach.

While the concept of social roles is self-explanatory, the developmental task concept may not be as commonly understood. A developmental task is affected by three possible forces, according to Havighurst. The forces are (1) biological development; (2) social demands and expectations; and (3) personal ambition and aspiration. Developmental tasks are set in childhood primarily by the first two forces while the last two forces dominate in adulthood. However with increasing senescence, the biological changes may probably be seen as again asserting a major force in setting and defining developmental tasks.

From ages twenty to forty, according to Havighurst, the individual seeks, establishes, and marshals his energies in solidifying his social identity. From ages forty to sixty, the individual progresses from increasing activity and assertiveness of self to maintaining activity and changing social roles. The decade after age sixty may focus on the process of disengagement and whether it should be undertaken. Social disengagement is a process whereby the individual decreases his interaction with others and becomes less socially active than he was previously. Psychological disengagement is a process whereby the individual decreases his emotional involvement, cares less for social approval, and tends to favor immediate instead of postponement of satisfactions. After age seventy, the developmental tasks center on completing formulation of a new and final pattern of restricted engagement or selective disengagement which may be satisfying for the individual.

In adult education as a whole, the forty- to sixty-year-olds have posed a problem of lacking motivation for education. By age forty, many have dropped out of adult education activity and new students are difficult to find. However, this is not the case in nursing. One of the new participants in continuing nursing education as well as in adult education is the woman who wishes to ready herself for employment after her children are grown. Since the large majority of nurses are women, nurse mothers with children nearing adulthood may be seen as a distinct advantage in recruitment of clientele for continuing education in nursing. Yet the realization also demands responsible recognition of the middle-aged nurse learner as more than merely a potential addition to the manpower pool. A refresher course is an obvious form of instrumental education for the nurse who plans to return to the practice of nursing. Yet expressive aspects of education, which may provide intrinsic satisfactions to the learner as the learning process goes on, need inclusion. For this reason the clinical component is as valuable as the theoretical framework of cognitive content in a refresher course.

Among the researchers investigating changes or phases during life, Erikson has been prominent. Well known in the fields of child development and psychoanalysis, he has identified eight ages of man with a tie at each stage between individual man and basic elements of society.[16] Although Havighurst and Erikson vary widely in their definitions of changes, a commonality of beliefs is seen in their views on how the influence of the degree of progress in a prior phase will affect achievement in later development. Thus, the better the teacher is able to assess where the learner is in relation to the learning which is to be undertaken, the greater is the likelihood for some success.

From the foregoing discussion, which has dealt with many factors and concepts affecting each individual learner, follows a consideration of assumptions that are useful to the teacher in guiding learning. The teacher in continuing nursing education confronts the reality of implications inherent to those assumptions.

ASSUMPTIONS AND IMPLICATIONS FOR LEARNING

Whether the nursing content to be taught is of a theoretical, affective, or psychomotor nature, the teacher who is able to value the uniqueness of each nurse learner is in a position to guide meaningful learning. Meaningful learning depends on the integration of the new and the old within the individual and a restructuring of knowledge as an outcome of additions, deletions, and revisions. In other words, learning must be relevant to the individual and he must be ready to learn. It is a personal experience with consequence for the individual. For example, when the nurse learns to identify and cope with common effects of anxiety, his nursing situation may improve through either his own or his patient's reduction of anxiety. Even when immediate application of new knowledge is not possible, gains may ultimately provide increased satisfaction. For example, the staff nurse may learn about the personnel appraisal conference at one time and the circumstances may be such that an actual appraisal conference is not scheduled until much later. Yet, the deferment of action may have added to the potential productivity of the conference.

REASONS FOR LEARNING

Every nurse learner is an independent adult who is responsible for his own choices and decisions. Even when attendance in a continuing education offering is required as a condition of employment, the nurse can exercise his options either to terminate his employment or to be inattentive and resist learning. Whether he learns or not is his personal decision. This does not absolve the teacher whose role will be discussed further in Chapter 7. However, the nurse as an adult learner is assumed to be as self-directing as any other adult in the society in which he lives. Thus, the implication is that the role of student may be viewed as one which may deprive the nurse learner of his autonomy as an adult. The relationship between teacher and student is ideally one of cooperative learning where each learns from the other rather than one being superior, and the other subordinate. A competent teacher draws upon the strengths of knowledge and experience which the nurse learner brings as a contribution to the teaching-learning process.

Because of varying kinds of preservice programs as well as a range of time since graduation and unique individual differences, nurses enrolled in many offerings demonstrate a diversity of levels in readiness to learn, interest, motives, and experiences. To provide points of contact to which every nurse learner may relate, the approach to content is most useful when previously acquired knowledge and past experiences of learners are acknowledged and shown to be related to the matter at hand. A forecast or summary of the study plan to be anticipated establishes a frame of reference for the class and serves as a guide in relating past, present, and future learning. Any plan for learning demands the active participation and involvement of the learner for his personal investment.

ORGANIZATION OF CONTENT AND SEQUENCE OF STUDY

Fragmenting learning and integrating content are terms which have been used in nursing education without perhaps a clear understanding of their impact. According to which school of thought in educational psychology is being advocated, learning bit by bit may seem to be more desirable than to learn a general whole before analyzing what comprises the whole, or vice versa. The question of the one best method of approach has yet to be resolved and will continue to be investigated. However, one assumption that may be made is that people learn in different ways. Historically in nursing, there tended to be one right way to do things with the implication that any other way was categorically wrong. In continuing nursing education, as far as learning is concerned, the "you do it your way and I'll do it mine" idea ought to be encouraged.

Organization of content and sequence of study are important to the obtaining of grasp and mastery in learning. Yet, depending on the particular nurses or content in a class, the teacher will find it useful to maintain some looseness and flexibility in arrangement of content. For example, if a class dealing with trends in health care is comprised of nurses who are instructors in hospital schools of nursing and the newspapers are reporting pending health legislation which may affect hospitals, hospital schools, and nursing students, benefit accrues to the learning process when the preordered plan is adjusted to relate pertinent aspects of content to current concerns in society with direct relevance to the class.

Learning is facilitated when new content is recognized as being different from present knowledge which the learner has. Opportunity is provided to help the learner examine some of the differences, make comparisons, and study the relationship between the old and the new. In a sense, relating new knowledge to previously acquired knowledge suggests that learning should proceed from the simple to the complex. But the definitions or criteria for simple and complex are not easily derived. For example, is headache as a symptom a simple or complex matter? When the difference between old and new material depends upon one clearly identifiable factor which is easily distinguishable, discrimination is simplified. The task of discrimination may become more difficult because of a complexity of factors which are not readily distinguishable as entities. Ease of discrimination may be a factor to consider in progressing from simple to complex organization and sequence of content.

If the nurse is learning to learn, the responses to instruction may be quite different for that individual compared to the responses that one who is ready to learn content is able to make. Instruction involves the learner and sequence is such that learners are provided opportunities to respond without being left out. The learner should not be expected to make a response when unable to do so. The nurse who is learning to learn may not be able to respond to a question calling for a critical analysis of a recent report when the act of reading such a report is the present extent of ability to respond to instruction. Thus, when the teacher develops the sequence of content, he must also consider abilities for response and encourage creative responses from the learners according to those abilities.

PRACTICE AND REINFORCEMENT

Practice as a term suggests action or involvement beyond an initial exposure to an idea. The purposes of practice are to facilitate understanding, to confirm learning, and to increase the retention of an idea through its use or application. While the concept of practice seems to enjoy a general acceptance among educational psychologists from varying schools of thought—the neobehaviorists and the Gestalt-field psychologists—the same cannot be said regarding the concept of reinforcement.

Reinforcement is directly related to a term which may be familiar to nurses, namely *operant conditioning.* Operant conditioning has been used as a therapeutic mode in working, for example, with autistic or mentally-retarded individuals as well as with some psychiatric patients. Reinforcement and conditioning are crucial to the learning process as perceived by neobehaviorists who may be defined as stimulus-response associationists. Gestalt-field or cognitive-field psychologists view the development of insight on the part of the learner as the crucial element of learning. From the latter's view, reflective learning and its improvement is of greater importance than the reinforced teaching promoted by the neobehaviorists.

In reinforcement and operant conditioning, the focus is usually on the response which the learner makes, and concerns the tendency of a future response to be affected by the feedback of reinforcement provided to the learner following the initial stimulus and response. The term *operant* refers to the operation or behavior which is the desired goal, outcome, or response. *Conditioning* refers to the response modified, changed, or different from the initial response and brought forth by a later substitute or conditioned stimulus. Again the response itself is not strengthened but the tendency to make the response is. In operant conditioning, the nature of the stimulus which elicits the initial response is not as important as the immediate presentation of the reinforcer after the initial response is made. The presentation of reinforcement may be made in a variety of ways—verbally, affectively, or materially. The reinforcer is the specific content or means used—the phrase "very good," a smile, or a blue ribbon.

Reinforcers, then, may be absent or present. If reinforcers are absent, a response may become extinct because the learning environment was not modified in any way following the response. If reinforcers are present, they may be either positive or negative reinforcers. Positive reinforcers add to the environment in some way, thereby modifying the circumstance. Negative reinforces take away something from the environment, thereby modifying the circumstance. Whether reinforcers are positive or negative, they are thought to strengthen the behavior on which conditioned stimuli depend.

In contrast, punishment is thought to weaken behavior on a temporary basis, unpredictably and undependably. Furthermore, punishment is not constructive; thus, extinction is a more desirable way to break habits than punishment which may take the form of sarcasm, ridicule, or embarrassment.

Reinforcement is provided by means of a feedback mechanism which the teacher may vary according to the learner and needs to be provided on a consistent basis. The learner needs not only to do a given task, but also to achieve the desired level of competence in his behavior. To attain retention of learning, reinforcement is required. Without reinforcement, extinction of learning may occur. For example, let us say that the nurse is learning content relating to shock and is presented with the facts concerning the causes of shock, such as cardiac inefficiency, loss of blood volume, and collapse of the vascular vessels. Unless these concepts are extended and related to specific or new situations to provide practice and reinforcement through application, learning may be temporary or limited in depth and retention. In addition to obtaining practice and reinforcement of learning, the adult learner as a self-directive person benefits from those opportunities which allow for his own sense of discovery and assessment of knowledge gained.

PARTICIPATORY LEARNING

Just as the nurse is recognized as a person with a background in nursing, the adult learner is recognized as a person with a background in learning. Thus, that resource of learning abilities needs to be guided and encouraged to develop further. Ways to engender participation on the part of the learner are to stimulate thinking, seek ideas, consider relationships of concepts, and encourage independent discoveries. Another way is to provide guidance in the process of self-evaluation whether the task of learning involves skills of problem solving or psychomotor activities. In fact, in learning anything, the process is likely to be as important for the adult as the content.

In terms of nursing, this means the nurse will learn who is an active participant in evolving the learning tasks, is involved in the learning process itself, and is able to resolve for himself the success of his learning. However, unless the teacher in continuing nursing education has predesigned plans for such participation, it is not automatically bound to happen. Planning for participatory learning is equally important for the nurse learner, the teacher, and the administrator in continuing nursing education.

Notes

1. Burton W. Kreitlow, "Part 1. Concepts for the Curriculum," *Educating the Adult Educator*, College of Agriculture, The University of Wisconsin, Madison, 1965, pp. 5-6.

2. J. R. Kidd, *How Adults Learn*, Association Press, New York, 1959, pp. 76-81.

3. Irving Lorge, "The Adult Learner," *Psychology of Adults*, Adult Education Association of the U.S.A., Washington, D.C., 1963, pp. 1-2.

4. Edmund deS. Brunner, David S. Wilder, Corinne Kirchner, and John S. Newberry, Jr., *An Overview of Adult Education Research*, Adult Education Association of the U.S.A., Chicago, 1959, p. 9.

5. Ibid.

6. Lorge, op. cit., p. 6.

7. Brunner, op. cit., pp. 29-31.

8. Raymond G. Kuhlen, "Motivational Changes During the Adult Years," in Raymond G. Kuhlen (ed.), *Psychological Backgrounds of Adult Education*, Center for the Study of Liberal Education of Adults, Boston, 1963, pp. 77-113.

9. Howard Y. McClusky, "The Relevance of Psychology for Adult Education," in Gale Jensen, A. A. Liveright, Wilbur Hallenbeck (eds.), *Adult Education: Outlines of an Emerging Field of University Study*, Adult Education Association of the U.S.A., Washington, D.C., 1964, p. 159.

10. Howard Y. McClusky, "An Approach to a Differential Psychology of the Adult Potential," in Stanley M. Grabowski (ed.), *Adult Learning & Instruction*, ERIC Clearinghouse on Adult Education and Adult Education Association of the U.S.A., Syracuse, 1970, pp. 82-83.

11. Howard Y. McClusky, "Course of the Adult Life Span," in Wilbur C. Hallenbeck (ed.) *Psychology of Adults*, Adult Education Association of the U.S.A., Washington, D.C. 1963, Chap. 2, pp. 15-18.

12. Abraham H. Maslow, *Toward a Psychology of Being*, 2d ed., Van Nostrand Reinhold Company, New York, 1968.

13. Ibid., p. 153.

14. Ibid., pp. 154, 211-212.

15. Robert J. Havighurst, "Changing Status and Roles During the Adult Life Cycle: Significance for Adult Education," in Hobert W. Burns (ed.), *Sociological Backgrounds of Adult Education*, Center for the Study of Liberal Education for Adults, Chicago, 1964, pp. 17-38.

16. Erik H. Erikson, "Eight Ages of Man," *Childhood and Society*, 2d. ed. rev. and enl., W. W. Norton and Company, Inc., New York, 1963, Chap. 7, pp. 247-274.

REFERENCES

Bigge, Morris L.: *Learning Theories for Teachers*, Harper and Row, Publishers, New York, 1964.

Brunner, Edmund deS., David S. Wilder, Corinne Kirchner, and John S. Newberry, Jr.: *An Overview of Adult Education Research*, Adult Education Association of the U.S.A., Chicago, 1959, p. 9.

Havighurst, Robert J.: "Changing Status and Roles During the Adult Life Cycle: Significance for Adult Education," in Hobert W. Burns (ed.), *Sociological Backgrounds of Adult Education*, Center for the Study of Liberal Education for Adults, Chicago, 1964, pp. 17-38.

Kidd, J. R.: *How Adults Learn*, Association Press, New York, 1959, pp. 76-81.

Klausmeier, Herbert J., and William Goodwin: *Learning and Human Abilities: Educational Psychology*, 2d ed., Harper and Row, Publishers, New York, 1966.

Kreitlow, Burton W.: "Part 1. Concepts for the Curriculum," *Educating the Adult Educator*, College of Agriculture, The University of Wisconsin, Madison, 1965, pp. 5-6.

Kuhlen, Raymond G.: "Motivational Changes During the Adult Years," in Raymond G. Kuhlen (ed.), *Psychological Backgrounds of Adult Education*, Center for the Study of Liberal Education of Adults, Boston, 1963, pp. 77-113.

Lorge, Irving: "The Adult Learner," *Psychology of Adults*, Adult Education Association of the U.S.A., Washington, D.C., 1963.

Maslow, Abraham H.: *Toward a Psychology of Being*, 2d ed., Van Nostrand Reinhold Company, New York, 1968.

McClusky, Howard Y.: "An Approach to a Differential Psychology of the Adult Potential," in Stanley M. Grabowski (ed.), *Adult Learning & Instruction*, ERIC Clearinghouse on Adult Education and Adult Education Association of the U.S.A., Syracuse, 1970, pp. 82-83.

McClusky, Howard Y.: "Course of the Adult Life Span," *Psychology of Adults*, (Wilbur C. Hallenbeck, editor) Adult Education Association of the U.S.A., Washington, D.C., 1963, Chap. 2, pp. 15-18.

McClusky, Howard Y.: "The Relevance of Psychology for Adult Education," in Gale Jensen, A. A. Liveright, Wilbur Hallenbeck, (eds.), *Adult Education: Outlines of an Emerging Field of University Study*, Adult Education Association of the U S.A., 1964, p. 159.

Melton, Arthur W. (ed.): *Categories of Human Learning*, Academic Press, New York, 1964.

Skinner, B. F.: *The Technology of Teaching*, Meredith Corporation, New York, 1968.

Staats, Arthur W., and Carolyn K. Staats: *Complex Human Behavior: A Systematic Extension of Learning Principles*, Holt, Rinehart and Winston, New York, 1964.

Symonds, P. M.: "What Education Has to Learn from Psychology: I. Motivation," *Teachers College Record*, 56 (February): 277-285, 1955.

Thorndike, E. L.: *Adult Learning*, The Macmillan Company, New York, 1928.

6

Planning for continuing education

Planning is the keystone to the administrative process. Without adequate planning, continuing education offerings are fragmented, haphazardly constructed, and often unrelated. A successful continuing education program is the result of careful and detailed planning.

Whatever the field of endeavor, planning for continuing education includes two major aspects: broad planning by institutions and agencies responsible for continuing education, and specific planning by individuals for their own continuing education. All too frequently there is too little planning involved in either instance.

Planning is essential if learning needs of nurses are to be met and if available resources are to be used to good advantage. Effective planning is required at all levels: local, state, regional, and national—and eventually international—to avoid duplication and fragmentation of efforts and to help keep at a minimum any gaps in meeting the continuing education needs of nurses.

In recent years there has been a proliferation of isolated activities provided by various special interest groups, resulting in a wide range of unrelated offerings available to nurses. These offerings are characterized by a lack of coordination of one activity with another, so that little or no continuity is provided to the learner.

Individual nurses may participate in a smattering of disconnected courses, and may enroll because the employing institution is willing to give him duty time or pay his expenses to attend or both. Many nurses appear to have given little attention to determining their own learning needs, but even if they had, counselling opportunities to assist them in the process are usually not available.

The increasing demands by nurses for continuing education have led to the provision of course offerings by many agencies, organizations, and institutions. Programs may be planned without serious consideration of educational objectives, and the selection of teaching faculty may depend upon the availability of the person rather than his expertise or teaching ability. The content of the program is designed around faculty knowledge rather than with reference to identifiable learning needs of the participants.

Frequently such offerings are of the "sit-and-listen" variety with little recognition given to the many factors involved in learning. Too often, a program is designed as a series of lectures by physicians with little, if any, time for questions or discussion. These lectures are usually illustrated with slides which may only remotely be related to the topic. Since the speaker's time is limited and he has a large number of slides to work through, it is not possible to explore the concept illustrated in depth. If any time is to be devoted to the nursing aspects of the content, it is scheduled for the end of the day, but unfortunately many of the participants have to leave early.

The above description is obviously not unique to nursing, but is generally typical in major areas of endeavor. Increasingly more thought, time, effort, and money are being diverted to planning on local, state, and regional bases. Such planning is imperative to avoid duplication of effort, to ensure that necessary services and quality education is provided to all who require them, and to assure the best utilization of available resources, including faculty.

Increasing attention is being directed to statewide planning for continuing education in nursing. Regional planning for continuing education in nursing dates back to 1957, with the Western Council on Higher Education for Nursing (WCHEN), followed shortly by the Southern Regional Educational Board. The Midwest Continuing Professional Education for Nursing (MCPEN) is comprised of eight states, and planning in other regions is underway. Some efforts along this line have been promoted by regional medical programs.

Enterprising commercial firms are becoming involved in various aspects of continuing education. Original interest was in the development of educational media, both hardware and software, but some firms offer various types of conferences for nurses and other groups. The quality of these offerings vary and, again, programs are sporadic, unplanned and unrelated to other educational endeavors.

The increasing emphasis on interdisciplinary approaches to continuing education calls for a different type of planning. Effective planning requires representation of all the groups involved. Too often interdisciplinary continuing education is seen as one group providing a program for another. The various health-related groups have different goals and priorities, so effective planning requires a determination of common and compatible goals for successful programming.

Another significant aspect of planning is that which is done by the learner himself for his own continuing education. This is discussed in detail in Chapter 12.

Planning must be seen as an ongoing process, not something that is done once for all time. The rapid technologic advances and proliferation of knowledge demands continuous planning to meet ever-changing learning needs.

THE PLANNING PROCESS

Nurses identify most closely with planning for patient care, but the principles of planning apply to a wide variety of situations. Various approaches may be used in planning for continuing education. A consideration of the elements in the planning formula (Exhibit 6.1) may be a useful approach since it identifies the significant aspects of planning, applicable to an overall continuing education program, as well as to any one specific activity.

The recent emphasis on management by objectives (M.B.O.) in industry and other agencies indicates the value now placed on the identification of significant organizational goals. These goals help determine priorities for the organization, allocation of effort and budget, and focus the workers' attention on expectations of the organization.

Another recent emphasis on planning can be seen in the establishment in many universities of graduate programs in city planning, health planning, and so on. A lack of planning in significant areas of daily life has resulted in devastating problems; planning for the future is essential to survival.

Whether planning broadly for continuing education or planning for one's own continuing education, the process is similar (see p. 200). The steps in the planning process are:

1. Establishing goals compatible with the purpose or mission of the organization.
2. Deciding upon specific objectives consistent with these goals.
3. Determining the course of action required to meet the specific objectives.
4. Assessing available resources for establishing the program; people and financial resources are of particular significance.
5. Establishing a workable budget, appropriate for the program.
6. Evaluating the results at stated intervals.
7. Reassessing the goals and updating the plan periodically.

Defining Purposes

Organizations have missions or purposes which identify their reason for existence. Educational institutions have very broad statements of purpose, into

Exhibit 6.1 THE PLANNING FORMULA

(The planning formula provides a framework for program planning.)

1. **WHAT IS TO BE DONE?**
    Get a clear understanding of what your unit is expected to do in relation to the work assigned to it. Break the unit's work into separate jobs in terms of the economical use of the men, equipment, space, materials, and money you have at your disposal. Think each job through.

2. **WHY IS IT NECESSARY?**
    When breaking the unit's work into separate jobs, think of the objective of each job. This may suggest alternate methods, or the possibility of eliminating parts of jobs or whole jobs. The best way to improve any job is to eliminate unnecessary motion, material, etc.

3. **HOW IS IT TO BE DONE?**
    In relation to each job, look for better ways of doing it in terms of the utilization of men, materials, equipment, and money.

4. **WHERE IS IT TO BE DONE?**
    Study the flow of work and the availability of the men, materials, and equipment best suited to doing the job.

5. **WHEN IS IT TO BE DONE?**
    Fit the job into a time schedule that will permit the maximum utilization of men, materials, equipment, and money; and the completion of the job at the wanted time. Provisions must be made for possible delays and emergencies.

6. **WHO SHOULD DO THE JOB?**
    Determine what skills are needed to do the job successfully. Select or train the man best fitted for the job.

Note: It is not always necessary to follow the steps in the order given above. Circumstances may cause changes in the order.

(Developed by the staff, Management Institute, University of Wisconsin Extension. Used with permission.)

which continuing education usually fits very well. Hospitals and related institutions also have broad purposes related to patient care, treatment, and research; the in-service education program can also be justified in terms of these purposes.

This broad statement of purpose gives direction in planning. An example of one such statement is the mission statement of University Extension, University of Wisconsin:

> . . . To bring to bear on the problems and interests of the citizens of the State all the available resources of knowledge, experience, teaching, demonstration and research which exist within the University Extension; to constantly strive to improve and expand Extension capacities in these areas; to serve as a channel through which the resources of the whole University can be made available to all State citizens and groups; to respond to specific requests for service from within the State; to initiate programs and activities which in the considered judgment of the initiators may meet unexpressed needs and interests; and to make Extension resources and capacities available to the citizens of this country and the world.

Out of this mission statement, the faculty in continuing education in nursing established the statement of purposes for the Department of Nursing in that organization:

> The overall objective of the Department of Nursing is to provide educational opportunities for the nurse and to encourage the continued learning and development of the individual. The major educational efforts are designed to enhance the competency of the learner to improve nursing care provided to the people of the State. Nursing care includes the promotion of individual and community health and the teaching of the patient and his family, as well as the care of the ill.

These broad statements of purpose assist the faculty in the determination of appropriate goals and in establishing priorities. Statements of purpose change as the needs of society change so are reviewed from time to time and restated as appropriate.

Establishing Goals and Objectives

Planning involves moving toward goals that are significant and realistic. Broadly defined, a goal is a state of affairs to be attained. Goals serve to stimulate and direct action and should be reachable, even though it may not be possible to determine the time at which attainment may be expected. Both short-range and long-range goals may be identified.

The terms *goal* and *objective* are often used interchangeably, but objectives are seen as more specific than goals. An objective is a desired end or accomplishment to be sought. An objective is quite specific in terms of things to

Exhibit 6.2 OBJECTIVES OF THE DEPARTMENT OF NURSING,
UNIVERSITY EXTENSION, UNIVERSITY OF
WISCONSIN

(Broad statements of objectives assist in setting priorities
for program planning.)

1. To assist the nurse in identifying and meeting current learning
   needs and those needs generated by changing professional
   practice.

2. To encourage the nurse to identify and influence societal changes
   which have implications for nursing and to modify practice
   accordingly.

3. To promote the development of leadership potential of the nurse.

4. To assist the professional nurse in identifying nursing problems
   and in seeking solutions to them.

5. To experiment with and develop varied teaching methods for
   extending nursing knowledge and competency.

6. To disseminate new information from the body of nursing
   knowledge and the health sciences through a variety of channels.

7. To facilitate and encourage the exchange of ideas and
   information among nurses.

8. To assist the nurse in systematically planning and pursuing
   continuing education.

9. To assist the nursing educator in increasing teaching effectiveness.

10. To promote a means for the nonpracticing nurse to relate to
    nursing and/or to facilitate a return to practice.

11. To provide a means of development for the nurse in-service
    educator to plan, implement and evaluate educational programs
    in hospitals and health facilities.

12. To conduct pertinent studies in nursing, particularly those
    relating to the continuing education of nurses.

13. To participate in the identification of health needs of citizens and
    to work with consumers as well as other health disciplines to
    meet these needs.

14. To seek opportunity for and collaborate with other health
    disciplines to effect improvement in the delivery of health care
    systems.

(continued)

Exhibit 6.2 CONTINUED

15. To maintain a liaison with the University of Wisconsin Schools of Nursing and the nursing service department of the Center for the Health Sciences.

16. To encourage and to provide opportunities for the continuing education of department faculty members.

Exhibit 6.3 CONFERENCE ON HEALTH MAINTENANCE ORGANIZATIONS: CONCEPT AND FUNCTIONS

(These examples of objectives for one type of educational activity, a conference, are stated as learner objectives.)

Specific objectives for the conference are to develop:

1. Knowledge of the health maintenance organization in evolution as a health care delivery concept and its functions in preventing and treating illness.

2. Understanding of evolving and changing roles of health professionals in going from a traditional system to a health maintenance organization system.

3. Understanding of the implications for nursing education and nursing services in the concept of health maintenance.

---

be accomplished and the time in which these are to be done. Objectives are usually established for an overall continuing education program, and are compatible with the purpose or mission of the organization. Objectives are also determined for any specific activity within that program. An example of the objectives of one continuing education program is given in Exhibit 6.2; objectives for one specific activity are illustrated in Exhibit 6.3.

Perhaps a mundane example will help clarify the difference between goals and objectives. We could say that a shopping list is an example of objectives for a shopping trip; without such a list, the shopper forgets to buy certain needed items. In addition she may find a bargain which is so enticing that she buys it, but in doing so spends the money intended to pay the gas bill. The shopper has not met her objectives, either because they were not identified or because they were ignored (she forgot to take her list with her). As a result she will have difficulty in meeting a family goal, that of balancing the budget.

Goal-setting is an important aspect of planning, and when determining goals, it is best to think broadly. Too many groups spend an inordinate amount of time in semantic arguments about the wording of specific goals or objectives, rather than upon the accomplishments to be attained.

DETERMINING NEEDS AND PRIORITIES

The accurate determination of learning needs and the establishment of priorities may well be the most neglected aspects of program planning. They are also most difficult and challenging aspects.

Without adequate assessment of needs, too much emphasis may be placed on occasional and isolated learning experiences. This results in a lack of continuity for the individual learner and in the provision of unrelated educational experiences.

The responsibility for determining needs and priorities varies from one state or region to another. In some instances it may be the responsibility of one agency or institution. In others, it may be the responsibility of a coordinating group. In the latter instance all the agencies and organizations involved in program planning are ideally represented on this coordinating group.

Assessment of Need

Attempts at assessment of needs have been made in a variety of ways. Surveys of various kinds have provided helpful information. These are often conducted in the form of mailed questionnaires or, less frequently, as personal interviews. With the assistance of experts in conducting surveys and through the use of computers, it is now possible to secure accurate information in a relatively short time.

Sample surveys may be meaningful, particularly if an adequate sample is selected and if random selection and assignment are used. The size of the sample must be large enough for drawing valid conclusions and must represent the various settings in which nurses are employed. Geographic representation is necessary for regional or statewide planning. It is erroneous to base program planning for one area on conclusions drawn from survey findings from an entirely different one.

Extensive surveys are time-consuming and costly, so there may be a temptation to use the data after it becomes outdated. Learning needs can change rapidly, so some means of updating data is required for effective program planning.

Feedback from participants in various courses can also provide clues to learning needs. These may be elicited from open-ended questions on course evaluation forms, or by specific check lists which enrollees are asked to complete. Informal discussions with individual participants, members of advisory committees, and others may assist in the identification of learning needs.

To a limited degree, spontaneous requests can also help identify needs. Some flexibility in program planning permits meeting these learning needs as they arise. This approach to need identification is limited, however, since not all nurses have the motivation nor the aggressiveness required to express their concerns.

Program planners must be alert to current and future developments in nursing and the health care fields. Keeping in mind Whitehead's admonition that "knowledge reduced to the level of practice results in stagnation," some planning must focus on future practice. Program decisions must be based on anticipated developments and not limited to the immediate needs identified by the learners themselves.

Future-oriented planning places great demands on planners, and requires many approaches for keeping alert to current trends and developments. A wide exposure to many different groups of nurses and allied professionals is useful, as is keeping up with the current literature.

Establishing Priorities

After an accurate determination of learning needs is obtained, the next step in the planning process is the ordering of priorities for meeting them. This may also be a challenging task, for the scope of nursing practice is so broad that many factors must be considered.

Since duplication of efforts is wasteful and costly, educational institutions ought not to offer those learning experiences that can better be provided by hospital in-service programs. But how to assist those nurses working in hospitals and other agencies that have little or no provision for inservice education?

With increasing emphasis on interprofessional continuing education, should a high priority be given to these efforts? Although most continuing education programs are designed for practicing nurses, what attention should be directed toward those nurses who are temporarily inactive? What priority should be given to programming designed for meeting future, in contrast to immediate, learning needs?

Another possible approach is placing the highest priority on the provision of educational experiences for those who work with many nursing personnel: directors of nursing, supervisors, teachers, in-service educators. By focusing on nurses in leadership positions, the learning achieved has the potential of reaching many others.

The nurse who works alone, as in an occupational health, school health, or public health agency, has special learning needs, and the means for meeting them is rarely provided by the employer. Should the learning needs of these nurses be given a higher priority than others?

This discussion suggests several areas for consideration in the establishment of priorities. Educational resources—particularly prepared faculty and financial support—are limited, so using these resources wisely demands a careful determination of priorities.

Statewide planning groups in nursing are directing more attention to assessment of learning needs and the establishment of priorities. This should result in more effective program planning and the better use of available resources.

ASSESSING RESOURCES

Resources for continuing education are detailed in Chapter 13, so in this chapter discussion is limited to a consideration of the assessment of resources. Any type of planning involves a careful assessment of ways and means to meet the established program goals. Faculty, finances, and facilities may be seen as the major resources required for a continuing education program.

Planning for resources consists of two aspects: a broad survey of the major resources necessary to the total continuing education program, and a more detailed assessment for any specific course or activity. Planning involves deciding upon the resources necessary to the activity and then determining their availability.

Adequate financial support deserves early consideration. If the assessment indicates a lack of sufficient support from the educational institution, other resources must be sought. Financial support is considered in detail in the next section of this chapter, beginning on page 91.

Even with adequate financial support, an effective continuing education program cannot be launched without sufficient and appropriate faculty. Planners should be aware of the availability of potential faculty members. Whether for an overall program or for a specific course or activity, preliminary planning involves at least a cursory determination of possible faculty members and their potential contributions. Identification of the skills required by faculty is part of this assessment.

The selection of faculty for a continuing education program, including qualifications of teachers, is considered in the next chapter. Information more specifically related to ad hoc instructors may be found in Chapter 13.

Facilities are the third major resource. Adequate and appropriate facilities are required for the continuing education staff. The facility should provide easy accessibility for visitors; these faculty members are likely to have more outside contacts than most other faculty members of the school of nursing. Adequate office space assumes satisfactory furnishings and equipment. Depending upon the type of program offered, the continuing education department may require considerable storage space for equipment, supportive materials, and related items.

Facilities for continuing education also include the space and necessary equipment required to conduct offerings. In many instances the entire program may be presented in the institution's conference center (see Chapter 13). Suitable conference rooms may be available in the school of nursing facility; in some settings a number of rooms are designed for, and their use limited to, continuing education offerings. In other instances it may always be necessary to seek space in an outside facility.

Unless assistance in locating suitable facilities is provided by the educational institution, the nurse educator may find it useful to develop an appropriate list of these resources. A card file listing, with notations about the availability and suitability of the facility, is a useful reference. A similar listing may also be developed for other types of resources.

FINANCING CONTINUING EDUCATION

Adult education in the United States has not received widespread public support, with the exception of vocational education and agricultural extension programs. The accomplishments in these areas of endeavor are dramatic illustrations of the value of adequate funding. Efforts are now being directed toward promoting legislation to provide federal support of other types of adult education.

Even in tax-supported institutions, continuing education in nursing has not received the attention it deserves. This is largely the result of inadequate financial support, and is associated with the struggle of collegiate schools of nursing to secure a sound financial base. In the face of limited budgets, nursing faculties have given continuing education a low priority.

A viable continuing education program is impossible without sound financial backing. In the past much has been accomplished through aid of various types of grants and other funds, but it is apparent that such support is only temporary. A sustained program with long range as well as short-range goals requires a firm financial foundation. A commitment to continuing education by an institution is only evidenced by the provision of adequate financial support.

Budgetary arrangements vary considerably from one institution to another, but the continuing education budget ought to be established on the same basis as that of comparable programs such as graduate education in nursing. In establishing a continuing education budget the same budgetary items are considered: salary for faculty, administrative, and clerical staff; office space, office equipment and its maintenance; travel, supplies and other expenses. There may be differences in the amount of salary support for ad hoc and part-time instruction as well as the amount budgeted for travel.

Program Budgets

In a number of institutions a separate budget is required for each specific activity, and each individual offering is expected to be self-supporting. To do this the person responsible must ascertain all the anticipated costs of the offering.

Programs which are totally self-supporting usually have a flexible fee plan, so the fee for each offering may be different. The fee is set on the basis of the cost involved and the expected enrollment. If the actual enrollment is less than that required to meet expenses, the course will usually have to be cancelled, since there is no way to make up the deficit.

It is obviously very difficult to determine actual costs of some items, so the institution may set some predetermined costs which are charged against the budget of every course. This may cover items such as an allocation for administrative costs, use of conference rooms, and so on. Budgeting for every individual activity is time-consuming, and requires skill not only in handling the budget itself but also in forecasting enrollment.

Those institutions requiring individual budgets for each offering may permit the nursing department to retain any additional money accrued as a result of excess enrollment. This provides some leeway in planning. In other instances this money goes into the institution's general budget.

Many educational institutions do not require that each individual offering be self-supporting but may expect this of the total program; at the end of the fiscal year, the budget must balance. In a few other institutions the program may be required to be only a certain percentage self-supporting, the remainder being financed by other funds.

Where policies permit considerably more latitude and a separate budget for each offering is not required, the institution may have an established minimum fee rate. As an example, minimum Extension fees at the University of Wisconsin are set at $1.25 per instructional hour, plus a $1.25 registration fee for the course. (This fee represents an attempt to equate continuing education course fees with undergraduate course fees). For costly programs a higher fee may be charged, but faculty members may not set a fee lower than the minimum one unless an outside agency provides financial support for the course.

This type of financial arrangement permits much more flexibility than budgeting for each offering. It helps assure the provision of certain courses that might not otherwise be financially feasible, but which contribute substantially to the continuing education of nurses.

Flexible financial arrangements are justified and necessary, particularly in the tax-supported educational institution, to provide a comprehensive continuing education program. Many learning activities cannot be budgeted directly. For instance, telephone or other consultation provided to practicing nurses is an important and often time-consuming activity. The value of this service of the university to practicing nurses cannot be measured and so cannot be accurately budgeted, yet it can be one of the most useful contributions of the institution.

Support by Tuition and Fees

From the foregoing it can be seen that many continuing education offerings are funded through fees or tuition collected by the educational institution. Continuing nursing education programs are usually supported wholly or in part by these charges. In some instances it may be difficult to recover costs through fees; this is particularly true if costs are high and enrollment low.

The established policies of the institution are followed in determining fees. Although this may provide some flexibility in setting fees for programs, in some instances the rigidity of the policy regarding fees may be detrimental to getting sufficient enrollment to warrant offering the course.

Nurses are not always aware of the costs of education and may be reluctant to pay the established fee, even though it is in line with others offered by the educational institution. This is also true of some employing agencies.

Certain agencies may be able to charge low tuition fees because faculty for the offering are expected to donate their services. For the voluntary health agencies this may be a reasonable expectation, although in many instances it is all too obvious that donated services are not entirely satisfactory, and a better program might have resulted from seeking out and paying for faculty whose major qualification is more than a willingness to give time to the activity.

Fee Payment. Payment of fees and other costs are often provided by the nurse's employing agency. The amount and extent of this financial support varies considerably from one institution to another. Concern has been expressed by some nurses that decisions about this financial support are often made on the basis of the size of the fee or the length of the offering rather than on the quality of the program.

Evidence of financial support by employing agencies is documented in a 1963 study by the authors of this book. In an analysis of participants in institutes and conferences offered by the University of Wisconsin, we found that three-fourths of the enrollees had their fees paid by their employers.[1]

Evidence that nurses themselves will pay for their own continuing education is also documented in the study cited above. Over 62 percent of enrollees indicated a willingness to pay the fees and expenses for participating in the given program. With the improvement in their economic status, perhaps in the future nurses themselves will be even more willing to support their own continuing education.

To a marked degree arrangements for financial support by employing agencies for their staff members have been rather haphazard. Procedures vary from one agency to another; in some instances a specific amount is budgeted for continuing education each year. In others decisions are made on the spur of the moment, and funds are juggled to permit the nurse to attend.

In determining the nurse's eligibility for receiving financial support from the institution to participate in a continuing education offering, arrangements may be so flexible that anyone requesting aid is permitted to attend at the agency's expense, if funds are available. At the other extreme, some institutions never provide this type of financial support and may not even permit the nurse time to attend. In some agencies, only supervisory or top administrative personnel have their fees and expenses paid, and staff nurses, who can least afford it, must make their own arrangements. Such a policy discourages participation by those who may have urgent learning needs.

To get the most from its educational dollar an institution must establish a rationale for providing financial assistance to staff members wishing to participate in continuing education offerings. A definite plan would prevent the same persons who always receive permission and assistance from taking part in available offerings. Advance planning by both the individual and the institution is required to use available funds wisely.

Except for short-term traineeships provided by the federal government and some funds allocated by voluntary health agencies, scholarship assistance for continuing education in nursing is rare. Unless other ways of supporting continuing education become available, more scholarship funds will be needed in the future.

Grant Support

A high proportion of continuing education activities are financed through grants, often from the federal government, but also from private funding sources such as philanthropic foundations. Although he may have access to sources of assistance in locating and applying for these funds, the administrator in continuing nursing education needs to be skilled in what is popularly known as "grantsmanship."

Even if assistance is available in locating sources of funds and in developing proposals, the nurse administrator must know the elements of a good project proposal and have the ability to write it in a convincing way. Specific assistance in preparing the budget is particularly useful, but developing the proposal itself is the responsibility of the educator.

In seeking funds it is usually a good idea for the inexperienced to start with a small project. Funding errors, such as underestimating travel costs, can be more easily rectified in a small project than in a larger one. Much can be learned from the experience of developing proposals, managing funds, and conducting a small project, that can be applied to a more extensive plan.

Preliminary Investigation. Before any proposal is developed, much preliminary work must be undertaken. Unless the project is so large that it starts with a feasibility study to ascertain its need, funds are not usually available to support the necessary investigation required to develop a sound proposal. Either the institution itself must then support this activity, or the project proposer must devote personal time and attention to its development.

A good proposal demands a clear definition of the problem to be studied. In any continuing education proposal, the definition of the problem requires adequate investigation of learning needs as identified by the learners themselves.

The identification of learning needs is documented by specific data. A program designed for school nurses, for example, should indicate the potential audience, where they are located, how large a group is involved, and what proportion of the group can be expected to participate in the proposed project. Supporting data indicates how knowledge of learning needs was derived (questionnaire, interview, observation of nursing practice, concerns expressed by supervisory personnel, and so on.)

Substantiating data should include some indication of administrative support, such as statements by appropriate organizations or supporting letters by administrative personnel. Administrative support is absolutely essential; in the example cited above, unless released time is provided for school nurses to participate, the project will fail because those for whom the offering is designed cannot attend.

Projects often involve cooperating agencies, and the nature and extent of the cooperation needs to be clarified for all parties concerned. This clarification is part of the preliminary planning and includes detailed and specific arrangements. For example, one agency may provide space to house the project, another to release time for teaching faculty, and still another to provide computer services to assist in the collection of data. Support by several agencies may strengthen a proposal but must be carefully defined in advance of writing the proposal.

A review of the literature to search for supportive data or to give evidence that little has been done in the area under investigation often contributes to a project proposal. Items included in a list of related references as a result of the literature search should be carefully selected and screened for their usefulness.

Preliminary investigation usually includes exploring possible funding resources. It also includes securing guidelines from these agencies and studying the

Exhibit 6.4   A SAMPLE FORMAT FOR PROPOSAL PREPARATION

(This format would be appropriate except in instances where the funding source specifies another format.)

I.   Cover sheet should include

    A.   Name of project
    B.   One-paragraph summary of project (optional)
    C.   Name of funding source to which proposal is directed
    D.   Name and address of institution submitting project
    E.   Name of principal initiator and others involved in proposal preparation
    F.   Date of submission

II.   One-page proposal abstract (optional) (See Exhibit 6.6)

III.   Proposal narrative should include

    A.   Statement of objectives
        1.   Describe nature of problem
        2.   Document existence of problem with appropriate data
        3.   Describe existing efforts (if any) to solve problem or create opportunity
        4.   Define target group
        5.   State goals of project (include and emphasize innovative features and multiplier effect, if any)
    B.   Procedure
        1.   Describe phases or sequences of procedures
        2.   Describe work performed at each stage and duration
        3.   Show how work will be organized
        4.   Tell which personnel will handle each component of work
    C.   Facilities required
    D.   Resources that will be tapped
    E.   Evaluation procedures

IV.   Budget (See Exhibit 6.5)

V.   Budget narrative

(continued)

Exhibit 6.4 CONTINUED

    A. Fully explain each budgetary item

    B. Include criteria and data used to make estimates

    C. Show detailed breakdown of budgetary materails where appropriate

    D. Explain with particular care unusually large budgetary items

VI. Appendices

    A. Statement outlining qualifications of institution requesting funds

    B. Vitae of personnel involved (include chief financial officer)

    C. Supporting statements from proposed clientele

    D. Supporting statement from cooperating individuals or agencies

(University of Wisconsin-Extension. Used with permission.)

criteria carefully to determine if the proposed project meets the requirements of a given agency. Criteria vary from one agency to another and change from time to time, so it is important to study a current copy of these requirements.

It is often useful to prepare a brief abstract of the proposal to use as a basis for discussion with appropriate individuals and groups. This abstract need not be detailed, but it should be complete enough to give a clear idea of the intent of the project and to indicate how it will be conducted.

Advisory or planning groups can be helpful in any project, and the early involvement of the individuals comprising the group often results in a more adequately designed proposal than would otherwise be true. Effective advisory groups include those who have had experience in developing proposals as well as some representation from the learning group for whom the project is intended.

Writing the Proposal. After the problem has been identified, the substantiating data collected, and the guidelines studied, the proposal is ready to be written. Deadline dates must be adhered to when submitting proposals and should be set with consideration of the applicant institution's own requirements for getting proposals through all its necessary channels.

The proposal should be written as carefully and concisely as possible but must include enough detail so that reviewers have a thorough understanding of what the project intends to accomplish. The language of the proposal should be clear, with unfamiliar terms defined and professional jargon omitted.

Exhibit 6.5   SAMPLE FORMAT FOR BUDGET PAGE

Project Title

Project Period _____ to _____

Personnel Services

　　List all position titles such as director,
　　assistants, secretaries, consultants, etc. Give the
　　annual rates and percent of time on the project.
　　Include any projected increases in the salaries.
　　Funds may be needed for part-time help to
　　cover emergencies.　　　　　　　　　　　　　$_____

Supplies and Expenses

　　Itemize by major category such as:
　　　　Office Supplies
　　　　Duplicating services
　　　　Instructional material
　　　　Telephone
　　　　Reference books
　　　　Publications
　　　　Printing of forms　　　　　　　　　　　$_____

Equipment

　　List by major categories such as:
　　　　Office equipment
　　　　Duplicating equipment
　　　　Cost of maintenance agreement
　　　　Audio visual equipment
　　　　State whether equipment will be
　　　　　　purchased or rented　　　　　　　$_____

Travel

　　How many trips? Where? By whom? Cost
　　per trip? Include expenses necessary for
　　consultants. List separately travel for staff and
　　consultants.　　　　　　　　　　　　　　　$_____

(continued)

Exhibit 6.5 CONTINUED

Space Needs

Indicate amount of space needed and the
monthly rental. Depending on lease, may be
necessary to include costs for maintenance,
heat, light, insurance, etc. $_____

Other Costs

Insurance (health and accident, hospitalization,
   theft, etc.)
Fringe benefits (social security, retirement,
   etc.)
Miscellaneous $_____

Trainee Costs

Subsistence
Travel
Salary or stipends
Space for classes $_____

TOTAL $_____

(University of Wisconsin-Extension. Used with permission.)

A funding agency may require that a specific format be followed and may
also provide directions for completing the detailed forms. If a definite format is
not required, a general outline may be used. A suggested format, a budget page,
and a proposal abstract are given in Exhibits 6.4, 6.5, and 6.6 respectively.

Planning a budget appropriate for carrying out the objectives of the
project requires considerable skill. Available assistance should be used, for
budget experts can often detect items that can easily be overlooked by the
unsophisticated. Explanation of budget items is usually expected; this requires
careful estimates. Arithmetical errors should be avoided.

A well-written proposal includes information about the target group for
whom the project is intended, including its composition, some general descriptive information, and the expected size of the group. Responsibilities and
qualifications of the staff are also identified.

Program content is described in enough detail to give reviewers an understanding of its purpose and intent. Teaching methods, tools, and materials to be

used are also detailed. Evaluation procedures are a necessary part of any project and are outlined in as much detail as possible.

Supportive and explanatory material may be included as an appendix to the proposal. Items that might be included in the appendix are listed in Exhibit 6.4. A careful review of these materials will help assure that only necessary items are submitted.

It is often desirable to have several persons read and react to the final draft of a proposal before it is submitted. These reviewers may uncover points that were missed by the person developing the proposal or may offer suggestions for its improvement.

Exhibit 6.6   SAMPLE PROPOSAL ABSTRACT

(An abstract of a proposal should have a length of approximately two pages, double-spaced.)

Proposal title:

Submitted by:

Problem:

Objectives:

Procedures:

Timetable:

Budget total:

(University of Wisconsin-Extension. Used with permission.)

EVALUATION

A well-designed plan for continuing education in nursing includes planning for an evaluation of the effectiveness of the program. Evaluation of patient care has always been a challenge in nursing, and at best this appraisal has been sketchy and incomplete. Since evaluation of continuing education in nursing relates so closely to the improvement of patient care, it must be viewed in terms of changes in the provision of that care. Effective evaluation requires considerable thought and skill; planning for this activity should begin early.

To date, evaluation is probably the weakest part of most continuing education programs. Evaluation is a significant consideration, particularly when effectiveness and impact of the program is weighed against cost. Program evaluation is discussed in detail in the last chapter.

Notes

1, Cooper, Signe S., and May S. Hornback, "The Continuing Learner in Nursing," University Extension, University of Wisconsin, Madison, 1966, p. 44. This paper is a description of nurses enrolled in institutes and conferences offered by the University of Wisconsin Extension Division, Sept. 1, 1962, to Aug. 31, 1963.

REFERENCES

Boyle, Patrick G.: *The Program Planning Process with Emphasis on Extension*, National Agricultural Extension Center for Advanced Study, University of Wisconsin, Madison, 1965.

Cooper, Signe S. and May Hornback: "Profile of the Continuing Learner in Nursing," *Nurs. Outlook*, 14(12): 28-31, 1966.

Curtis, Frieda Smith, et al.: *Continuing Education in Nursing*, Western Interstate Commission for Higher Education, Boulder, Colorado, 1969, pp. 26-30.

Flaherty, Josephine: "An Enquiry into the Need for Continuing Education for Nurses in the Province of Ontario," Master's thesis, University of Toronto, Toronto, 1965.

Foerst, Helen, Florence E. Gareau, and Eugene Levine: *Planning for Nursing Needs and Resources*, Department of Health, Education, and Welfare Publication (NIH) 72-87, Washington, D.C., 1972.

Hornback, May: "The Nature and Extent of Inservice Program for Professional Nurses in General Hospitals in Wisconsin," Ph.D. dissertation, University of Wisconsin, Madison, 1969.

Houle, Cyril O.: *The Inquiring Mind*, The University of Wisconsin Press, Madison, 1961.

Kidd, J. R.: *Financing Continuing Education*, The Scarecrow Press, Inc., New York, 1962.

Lee, Barbara: "Financial Support for Continuing Education," *J. Contin. Educ. Nurs.*, 2(5): 7-12, 1971.

National Commission for the Study of Nursing and Nursing Education: *An Abstract for Action*, McGraw-Hill Book Company, New York, 1970.

Parelius, M. Ronald: "You Can Write a Good Grant Application," *Northwest Med.*, **68**(1): 52-54, 1969.

Price, Elmina Mary: *Learning Needs of Registered Nurses*, Teachers College Press, Teachers College, Columbia University, New York, 1967.

Professional Nurse Traineeships, U.S. Public Health Service Publication 1154-1, rev., 1969.

Schweer, Jean E.: "Critical Issues in Continuing Education in Nursing: Determining Needs and Priorities," *J. Contin. Educ. Nurs.*, **2**(4): 14-20, 1971.

Skinner, Geraldine: "What Do Practicing Nurses Want to Know?" *Amer. J. Nurs.*, **69**(8): 1662-1664, 1969.

Veri, Clive C.: "How to Write a Proposal and Get it Funded," *Adult Lead.*, **16**(9): 318-320; 343-344, 1968.

7

The teacher
in continuing education
in nursing

Of all the responsibilities of an administrator of a continuing education program in nursing, none is more important than the selection of faculty. This selection occurs at two levels: securing faculty members with a primary responsibility in the overall continuing education program, and locating appropriate teaching faculty for a specific activity. Although the considerations in selection apply to both, the emphasis in this chapter is on the teacher who has a faculty appointment.

The ad hoc faculty member is a person identified for a single presentation or a limited activity. He is often chosen primarily for his expertise in a given subject matter area rather than for his knowledge of the principles of adult education and his skill in applying them. If his lack of skill in working with adults places an added burden on the conference coordinator, his expertise contributes substantially to the content.

Although many of the principles of adult education can be applied to the teaching of late adolescent students, there are some basic differences in teaching the novice and in teaching those who come with practical experience. Also, at the present time there are major differences in the educational preparation of the registered nurse enrollees in many continuing education activities. Unless the teacher recognizes these differences and adjusts his teaching accordingly, he may expect difficulties, if not outright failure, in reaching the students.

Adult learners expect the teacher to identify with them on the problems they face in the world of work; these learners demanded relevance of content long before relevance became an undergraduate campus call to action. But education must consist of more than solving immediate problems. The teacher must help the learner discover new approaches and become excited about potential developments in his field. Thus the teacher walks a tightrope between the reality of today and the anticipation of tomorrow and the future.

ROLE OF THE TEACHER

In all areas of education, the role of the teacher is changing. From the traditional view of the teacher as a dispenser of wisdom and knowledge, the emerging view is that of the teacher as a guide in the learning process, assisting wherever appropriate, encouraging activities that promote learning, and stimulating and promoting individual thought.

The rapid advancement of knowledge has forced a recognition that a major role of the teacher is to help the student in learning how to learn, to face an uncertain and changing future. Perhaps this was best stated in the oft-quoted words of the anthropologist Margaret Mead:

No one will live all his life in the world into which he was born, and no one will die in the world in which he worked in his maturity. For those who work on the growing edge of science, technology, or the arts, contemporary life changes at even shorter intervals. . . . In today's world, no one can "complete an education."[1]

The skillful teacher is aware of the difference in learning what is already known and encouraging exploration in those areas yet to be discovered. Creative teaching in adult education is of crucial importance, for mature students enter a learning situation with a variety of work and other life experiences which contribute to and enhance learning. The effective teacher takes advantage of the assets which the learner brings with him.

In the past the teaching in schools of nursing focused on the cycle of conformity in education, that is, teaching what is already known. But the next cycle, creativity, which is seeking to find out what is yet to be discovered, is a more significant aspect of education. The ability to encourage students to move in this direction is the mark of the creative teacher.

In studies of teacher effectiveness, no clear-cut picture emerges of the effective teacher of adults. Different competencies are required of the teacher of adults than of the teacher of children, yet there seem to be a number of commonalities. Among these are the teachers' feelings towards his students—his humaneness.

The relationship of the teacher to his students in a mode that is conducive to learning is worthy of consideration. Student expectations vary, and obviously not every teacher can be successful with every student. The writings of Cantor, Rasey, Rogers, and others document the impact on learning of the relationship

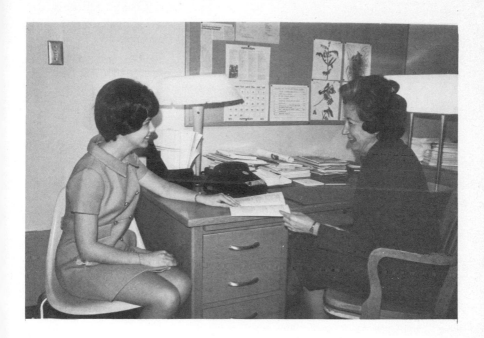

Figure 7-1   Counseling a potential continuing education student is an important role of the teacher. Effective counseling requires skill and adequate time, and must take place in a setting that assures privacy. (*Gary Schulz, University of Wisconsin-Extension*)

between the student and the teacher. A warm, helping, trusting relationship creates a climate that promotes learning. It is not improbable that this factor remains a significant one as learning progresses throughout life, though perhaps to diminishing degrees as the learner matures.

Whatever his area of expertise, the effective teacher shows his interest in and concern for every member of his class. He is able to instill in his students a sense of their own adequacy and the feeling of confidence in themselves so necessary to the learning process. Just how this is accomplished is difficult to identify and certainly varies between individual teachers and in different educational settings.

Every experienced educator is aware that he learns much from his students. This is illustrated in the lines of the Broadway musical, *The King and I*: "If you become a teacher, by your pupils you'll be taught." Because adult students come with a rich background of experience, they contribute much to the education of the teacher, and this two-way teaching-learning process is of great significance to nursing education. The teacher who leaves the large medical center to participate in a workshop where most of the enrollees come from small institutions may discover many nursing problems of which he is totally unaware. Recognition of these problems and, with the enrollees, seeking possible solutions, can contribute much to his overall understanding of nursing practice.

The continuing educator has a variety of roles to fill: as a guide and counselor to the learner, as an arranger and organizer of learning experiences, as an encourager and motivator of students, as an evaluator of programs. The specific role depends upon the setting in which the educator is employed. Thus, in the hospital the inservice educator may have a major role in involving others, particularly head nurses, in teaching the staff; in the university setting, the educator will do much of the teaching himself. Regardless of the setting, the role of the educator is a demanding and challenging one which may vary somewhat from day to day.

As part of the teaching function, the adult educator often has a role in the production of instructional materials, but he must also have the ability to select and evaluate materials prepared by others. The easy access to such materials places an increasing responsibility on the teacher for careful selection and appropriate use of materials. He also has a concomitant responsibility to be ever more sensitive to those unique human teaching activities which cannot be provided by educational technology.

In addition to his role as an instructor and counselor, the continuing educator usually has an administrative role in his institution, including participation in policy planning. These administrative responsibilities vary with the specific position but may include planning, directing, budgeting, and evaluation, all of which are discussed elsewhere in this book.

Public Relations

Every nurse educator—indeed, every nurse—has a public relations role in the interpretation of nursing. The nurse in continuing education often has a more extensive public relations role, simply because he is often with more people, both lay and professional, than many other nurses.

The public relations role is a broad and diffuse one and, as with many other roles of the teacher, will vary in the particular setting. Public relations activities may range from preparing news releases about a specific event to serving on community health planning committees.

As part of the public relations function, the continuing educator must be familiar with the many health-related organizations in existence today. This often involves working closely with the staffs of these organizations.

The adult educator often finds the public relations role a difficult and time-consuming one. Not many are prepared for these responsibilities and for the challenge of working with a variety of persons, each with a different background, point of view, and expectations. This public relations role may be of particular significance to nursing generally, for the nurse educator often has many opportunities to interpret nurses and nursing to the public. The nurse educator in continuing education needs an awareness of the significance of this role and its potential impact on the public in changing the image of nursing and in recognizing the contributions and potential of nurses.

EDUCATIONAL PREPARATION

In all of nursing education today, locating adequately prepared faculty is very difficult since educationally prepared nurses are in short supply. Selection of faculty members in continuing education is even more difficult, for relatively few nurses have any formal preparation for teaching adults.

Although educational requirements vary from one position to another, it would seem that the ideal preparation of the nurse educator in continuing education is a master's degree in his area of nursing expertise, with a doctorate in adult education. In most situations, compromise is necessary, but the academic preparation of faculty members whose major responsibility is continuing education ought to be at least the same as for any other nurse faculty member in the institution. There may even be a valid argument for expecting more preparation for the faculty member in continuing education, since in many instances he is working with experienced practitioners.

Information about the preparation of nurse educators in continuing education is limited but was explored by Betty Gwaltney in a survey reported at the 1969 National Conference on Continuing Education for Nurses. Of the 32 directors of continuing education programs who responded to the questionnaire, 27 held master's degrees, four had doctoral preparation, and one a baccalaureate degree. The majority of additional faculty members employed full time in continuing education held master's degrees.[2]

Less educational preparation may be expected of the in-service coordinator than of the educator who is a member of a college or university faculty, although this varies with institutions. Obviously the in-service coordinator should be better prepared than those he is attempting to teach.

It is common practice in many institutions to employ an available nurse, regardless of preparation, rather than seek the person most suitable for the requirements of the position. The difficulty in locating prepared nurses for in-service education positions has been identified by May Hornback in her study of in-service practices in Wisconsin Hospitals in 1968. At that time only 26 percent of in-service coordinators held a baccalaureate degree.[3] This was further documented in a study conducted by *R.N. Magazine* in 1971; 42 percent of those who responded to this survey held a baccalaureate degree, and an additional 10 percent had a master's degree.[4]

In assessing a candidate's credentials, consideration is given to the content of the curriculum he pursued, particularly as it relates to the job expectations. If his responsibilities are largely administrative, this should be reflected in his curriculum; if he is expected to do research, he needs appropriate preparation in this area.

The candidate's credentials will list his publications. Although some continuing education programs may not be hamstrung by a publish or perish tradition, the ability to write clearly is a significant faculty qualification, whatever the position. Continuing education may take many forms, most of which require the ability to speak and write effectively. Good writing demands clear thinking, meaningful organization of materials, and skill in putting one's ideas across. The quality of the candidate's publications provides some clues to these abilities.

OTHER QUALIFICATIONS AND COMPETENCIES

A variety of skills are required for the teacher in any educational program; these skills vary, depending upon the content to be taught, the potential students, the setting in which the learning occurs, and the specific responsibilities assigned to the faculty member. The selection of a faculty member obviously depends upon the requirements for the specific position. But whatever that position, there are some general qualifications that must be seriously considered for every applicant.

The Continuing Educator as a Continuing Learner

The candidate's acceptance of his personal responsibility for his own continued learning is a qualification of paramount importance. He must be what is sometimes described as a chronic learner. During the employment interview, one can determine the applicant's plan for this learning, his reading patterns, his participation in professional and other organizations, and his interest in additional appropriate learning activities. Although each person learns in his own way, it is helpful to determine the extent of his in-depth personal study and his awareness and use of available learning resources.

Recognizing that individuals learn at their own pace and in their own way, each candidate's plan for his own continued learning will be different. Some set aside a definite time each week for library study; others find it stimulating to discuss current issues and the nursing literature with a group of colleagues; still others find it helpful to listen to audiotapes or other verbal presentations; many learn from a combination of these approaches. The most significant factor is that a specific plan is made for self-development, and a definite time set aside for learning. Unless a plan is followed, other things take precedence in spite of good intentions.

Much is expected of the adult educator, but in an educational institution it is not unreasonable to expect that the teacher will be involved in some type of ongoing study or research in his area of expertise. The extent of this activity is limited by other responsibilities, but the need for research in continuing education is acute, and institutions must provide opportunities for this activity. In turn, faculty members must be prepared for this responsibility and be willing to accept it and to recognize its importance to their professional development.

It can be argued that the teacher's greatest contribution is to instill in students a zest for continuing to learn themselves. Thus the effectiveness of the teacher as a continuing learner role model deserves a high priority.

Clinical Knowledge and Skill

Clinical expertise is another significant attribute of the nurse educator in continuing education. To work effectively with nurses, faculty members must have a depth of nursing knowledge and skill in its application. Practicing nurses are quick to sense the difference between theoretical and practical knowledge, and clinical inadequacies may create an insurmountable "credibility gap." Nurses recognize that no nurse can be an expert in all areas of professional practice, but have the right to expect some depth of nursing knowledge and skill. The statement "Those who can, do—those who can't, teach" is a sad reflection on the state of some types of education, and is said of nursing faculty often enough to be of serious concern.

In the selection of a faculty member, an evaluation of the applicant's clinical experience is of primary importance, particularly as it relates to the expectations in the proposed position. The applicant's suggestions for retaining his clinical competence should be considered in the employment interview. It was suggested earlier that nurses in continuing education ought to have at least the same academic qualifications as other faculty members, but since this educator works with practicing nurses, perhaps more extensive clinical experience may be required of him than of other nurse faculty members in the same institution.

Clinical expertise suggests a depth of knowledge in the subject the candidate is expected to teach. Interest in the subject is enhanced by the teacher's enthusiasm for it. Is this enthusiasm contagious, so that students also develop an excitement about the subject?

Working with Adults

Skill in working with adult learners is another competency expected of the teacher. In continuing education programs in nursing, the faculty member may need special ability in working with groups, for learning groups in nursing may be quite heterogeneous, even with definite enrollment requirements.

It takes special skill to assist nurses in using the wealth of practical experience they bring with them. They need assistance in reformulating previously learned content and attitudes about patients and personnel. Special ability is required to help practicing nurses develop an awareness of or overcome reluctance to consider certain aspects of care, such as the care of the dying.

Skill is also required to help nurses feel comfortable in new teaching techniques. Traditional teaching in nursing has been of the lecture type, and many nurses feel quite uncomfortable with participatory approaches to learning, such as group discussions or role playing. Helping these nurses develop a willingness to attempt new approaches takes special skill and patience.

Broad Knowledge Base

In addition to clinical competence, the continuing educator needs an awareness of current developments in nursing and in the broad areas of health. Such an awareness includes an understanding of significant social and economic issues, current trends in nursing and medical practice, general educational trends, significant health legislation, and innovative developments in the delivery of health care.

The knowledgeable nursing educator is familiar with the major contributions of other members of the health team. He recognizes that along with nursing, other health professions are undergoing major changes that will affect the practice of all. A familiarity with these changes will facilitate interdisciplinary planning and programming. For example, if the nurse recognizes the pharmacist's role in health teaching as customers request over-the-counter drugs in the neighborhood drug store, he appreciates the need for more collaborative efforts in teaching about health.

Active participation in nursing and other organizations helps the nurse keep abreast of current professional concerns, but different approaches are required to keep current in other areas. This presupposes that the teacher reads broadly, listens to the radio or views television selectively, participates responsibly in community affairs, and keeps generally well-informed on citizen concerns.

The effective teacher is well-informed, and applies this knowledge of the world around him to his teaching. Relating nursing to current societal concerns keeps teaching relevant, and helps the nurse better appreciate his own need for a deeper understanding of these concerns. In teaching about emphysema, for example, one can hardly escape a consideration of air pollution and its serious consequences for health.

Concern for People

Working effectively with groups implies an understanding of and a concern for people as individuals. One expects nurses to possess a high degree of empathy and understanding of people, but it cannot be assumed that all nurses have this characteristic.

Students expect teachers to be seriously interested in them, but concern for students may be expressed in many ways. Obviously, not all students react positively to the effervescent teacher, particularly if they sense insincerity in the teacher's words. The shy, reticent teacher may have more appeal for some students, especially when they come to appreciate his other attributes.

Attending a conference may require that the nurse learner make considerable adjustment in family and job responsibilities. The person is often placed in an unfamiliar setting, with people he does not know; he may be reluctant to ask for assistance in areas that seem obvious to other participants. (The writer recalls one conferee who had never stayed at a hotel prior to attending the conference and was at a loss in making arrangements.) Genuine concern for participants and their needs—or lack of concern—may make the difference between a successful and an unsuccessful continuing education program.

Flexibility

Flexibility is another highly desirable trait for the teacher of adults. Perhaps in no other field than nursing is there such diversity in educational background, and perhaps in no other area of human endeavor do we expect so much of relatively short periods of training. This diversity places extra demands upon the teacher of the practitioners.

Program content requires adjusting to the needs of the specific learner, and a lack of recognition of these learning needs may result in untold frustration for both the student and the teacher. For example, the teacher may want to focus discussion on the nursing process, but the learners may be so troubled by more specific problems that they fail to learn from any consideration of the philosophical aspects of planning nursing care. At the same time the teacher must learn to recognize the point at which prolonged discussion of one student's peculiar problem may not be appropriate to the entire group and may lead to frustration for most participants. The skillful teacher is sensitive to group response, and makes necessary adjustments. Individual counseling may be more appropriate in dealing with specific problems of individuals.

The compulsive teacher may not feel comfortable unless every minute of the conference day is planned. In planning for adults, *allowing adequate time for exchange of ideas is basic.* This may provide the most satisfactory learning experience for some participants. Although this may have been a facetious comment, an enrollee in one meeting indicated that she felt the coffee break was the best part of that particular conference; the statement suggests that breaks of various types provide enrollees opportunities for learning from each other, possibly in areas where the teacher cannot assist them.

In contrast, some ineffective teachers use the opposite approach, permitting the discussion to go far afield. Since conference participants usually elect to enroll on the basis of content to be presented, such behavior is very distressing to many enrollees. Flexibility in presenting content is highly desirable, but changes must be made with discretion, based on sound judgment and valid reasoning.

Flexibility is a particularly important requirement for the off-campus teacher. The itinerant teacher may not find all the equipment he expected; can he still make his content meaningful and interesting without the slides he usually uses? Can he adapt to less than ideal physical facilities? No matter how carefully plans are made, adjustment may be required. Adult learners can be flexible if the teacher can adjust to the situation that presents itself.

Flexibility is required in working with colleagues and other faculty members. Rigid adherence to one's pet ideas can be detrimental to an effective continuing education program and damaging to peer relationships. Each faculty member must respect the opinions and beliefs of his colleagues and must possess a willingness to make appropriate adjustments in resolving differing points of view.

The continuing nurse educator must also be flexible in working with part-time or ad hoc faculty. Based on his own knowledge and experience, the adult educator may have firm convictions about the conduct and management of courses. He gives assistance and support as indicated, but he must recognize that the participating faculty member needs the opportunity to try out his own approaches. An acceptance of this concept is basic to academic freedom.

A successful continuing education program requires flexible faculty members. They must possess a willingness to adapt to the demands of the situation, placing the learner's needs ahead of their own and, when necessary, adjusting to the needs of other faculty members.

Creativity

The identification of creative individuals is often difficult, but this important attribute ought to have a high priority in the selection of faculty. Since continuing eduation programs in nursing are of relatively recent origin, at this time it seems particularly significant to select faculty members with the ability to develop imaginative approaches to continuing education.

Creativity may be expressed in many different ways. This factor alone may make its identification difficult. Some creative persons are at their best in working alone; many appear to be stimulated by modifying or adapting others' ideas. Freedom to work at one's own pace and method may foster creative thinking.

Creative faculty members are a challenge to the administrator of any program; they raise questions, disagree with traditional approaches, demand instant action. Today nursing is crying for creativity, and continuing education programs must accept this challenge.

The teacher with a questioning mind encourages this quality in his students. He must not be too ready to give out answers, regardless of pressures by students. Creating undue dependence upon the teacher may satisfy his personal needs but is an injustice to the student and defeats the major purpose of education: to help the student become a responsible, independent learner. The creative teacher can foster creativity in his students.

Other Characteristics

In the selection of faculty for any continuing education program, a number of other characteristics may be desirable. The relative significance of each may vary according to the specific position, but all are important enough to consider for any potential faculty member.

In almost any continuing education program in nursing, the faculty member must be willing to travel. This expectation may be greater in the state tax-supported educational institution, where off-campus teaching is usually part of the educator's responsibility. However, in any program the nurse educator must have the freedom to go out to nursing practice areas to discover for himself the problems faced by practitioners and to seek to identify their learning needs.

In addition to having a willingness to travel, the nurse educator needs the ability to organize for itinerant teaching. Long-distance planning places special demands on the teacher, including detailed advance preparation and organization for teaching. He must be able to anticipate the needs of the particular situation and have adequate teaching materials available for use.

Resourcefulness is a useful quality for an adult educator, since adaptation to students' learning needs and to a wide variety of teaching situations is often required. Resourcefulness and flexibility are often closely related: the flexible teacher usually knows how to make the most of available resources and existing circumstances.

In many educational settings, determination is a useful asset to the educator. Determination, self-confidence, and a firm belief in what one is doing help the teacher through difficult situations and give him the courage to try new ideas. Since experimental programs in continuing education are so badly needed, administration must give faculty members the right to fail, but failure is difficult for many teachers to accept. The mature teacher is more accepting, since he recognizes that learning can also result from failure.

A sense of humor appears to be another prerequisite for the successful adult educator. This characteristic helps the person through difficult and trying situations. Students appreciate this quality in teachers who skillfully use humor to add variety to their teaching or to ease tense situations.

Today's nurse practitioner has a broader outlook and a wider range of interests than was characteristic of nurses in the past. Several factors have contributed to this change: the shorter work week; a greater exposure to a wide range of educational and other life experiences; a familiarity with larger numbers of people, including those from different social and economic classes; an easier access to and a wide variety of opportunities which facilitate the development of broad interests. These opportunities provide the potential for nurses to develop interests in many different areas. Generalizations are unfair, but perhaps it can be said that as a result of all these contributory factors, nurses today are more interesting as people than was once true. This quality is important to the adult educator.

A zest for life, an innate curiosity, a love of adventure, a desire to search the unknown—all contribute to self-development. Since these qualities in nursing seem important to professional practice, they are especially significant to the teacher of the practitioner.

Today we recognize that we cannot expect students to treat patients as individuals unless they themselves are treated as such, so individuality is encouraged. It follows that continuing nursing educators of the future will have differing outlooks, various points of view, and a broad range of interests.

Obviously, each faculty member possesses different characteristics and competencies, and the strength of any faculty may very well rest with its diversity. Faculty members should be carefully selected to counteract each others' deficiencies and augment each others' strengths. By working in unity, they make the whole effort greater than the sum of its individual parts.

THE FACULTY ADMINISTRATOR

The nurse administrator of a program in continuing education must possess qualities comparable to those of the faculty he directs, particularly if teaching is part of his responsibility. In addition the director of the program must possess a high degree of administrative skill.

The skillful administrator assesses and uses the various abilities of different faculty members. He recognizes these differences as a strength of the program and aggressively searches for faculty with a wide variety of talents.

In the reality of today, with limited budgets and relatively few adequately prepared faculty members, the administrator may not always be able to employ the most talented people. At present, then, the administrator must devise means to help faculty members strengthen their teaching skills. Providing an adequate orientation, creating opportunities on the job which contribute to faculty growth, and encouraging supplemental education may all be seen as administrative responsibilities.

The provision of an environment conducive to promoting personal and professional development and encouraging creativity is an administrative responsibility. In such an environment, faculty members are free to raise questions, explore new concepts, and develop imaginative approaches to helping nurses meet their learning needs. The creative teacher is at his best in an environment which fosters the expansion of his talents.

It may be equally important to help faculty accept and carry out more mundane responsibilities which may be less satisfying to them, but just as urgent. Teachers may chafe against committee assignments, or argue that faculty meetings are a waste of time, or object to repeating certain courses, even in the face of obvious need. The effective administrator is aware of faculty impatience of these activities and strives for a balance between the routine and the more interesting, but helps teachers realize and accept their broad responsibilities as members of a faculty.

Working with an imaginative staff may challenge the administrator, but the results are rewarding. It may require unusual patience to work with the impatient instructor who wants instant action on all his ideas and concerns. Tolerance may be required for the intolerant teacher who cannot abide what he considers needless restrictions. Restraint may be necessary for the exuberant faculty member who wants to try everything he hears about.

Being a faculty member of an educational institution places demands on the individual for responsible action. Traditions and long-established patterns of behavior can be altered, but orderly change comes about best by concerted action. Faculty members must accept responsibility for helping the institution meet its goals and must learn how to work with colleagues to bring about desired changes.

Faculty members are expected to support and abide by institutional policies, but interpretation of these policies to faculty is the responsibility of the administrator, who must be thoroughly familiar with them. A lack of understanding of policies and procedures is wasteful of time and energy and causes unnecessary strain.

Administrative support to faculty occurs at various levels but is essential to an effective continuing education program. Adequate administrative support permits the maximum use of faculty time for those activities which only faculty can perform.

The effective administrator is prepared to meet the unexpected; if flexibility is a desired qualification of the faculty member, it is even more necessary for the director. Adjustments are required when a conference leader misses his plane, when delays in printing interfere with mailing of brochures, or when a blizzard is predicted for the opening day of a major conference.

The skillful administrator must guard against the interference of his own needs with the good of the program. He must support his faculty and accept responsibility—and sometimes blame—for errors in judgment, but must always be willing to share successes. Working together with an able administrator, the faculty knows that each made an important contribution to the total venture, and that each person's contribution is recognized and valued.

Notes

1. Margaret Mead, "A Redefinition of Education," *NEA Journal,* **48**(7): 16, 1959.

2. Betty Gwaltney, "Continuing Education in Nursing—Where We Are," *Proceedings Book, National Conference on Continuing Education for Nurses,* School of Nursing, Medical College of Virginia, Health Sciences Division of Virginia Commonwealth University, Richmond, Virginia, November 10-14, 1969, p. 24.

3. May Shiga Hornback, "The Nature and Extent of Inservice Programs for Professional Nurses in General Hospitals in Wisconsin," Doctoral dissertation, University of Wisconsin, Madison, Wisconsin, 1969, p. 71.

4. "Inservice Education, How it Really Is," *R.N. Magazine,* **34**(2): 39, 1971.

REFERENCES

Aichlmayr, Rita Hoescher: "Creative Nursing: A Need to Identify and Develop the Creative Student," *J. Nurs. Educ.,* **8**(4): 19-21; 24-27, 1969.

Brunner, Edmund deS., and William S. Nicholls II: "The Adult Educator: His Gratification, Problems and Hopes," *Adult Lead.,* **8**(7): 204-213, 1960.

Burt, Jesse: "Socrates May Have Been Right," *Adult Lead.,* **17**(9): 394-396, 1969.

Burton, William H.: *The Guidance of Learning Activities,* Appleton-Century-Crofts, New York, 1962.

Cantor, Nathaniel: *The Teaching-Learning Process,* The Dryden Press, New York, 1953.

Cooper, Signe S.: "The Development of Leadership in Nursing," *J. Contin. Educ. Nurs.,* **2**(2): 7-13, 1971.

de Tornyay, Rheba: *Strategies for Teaching Nursing,* John Wiley and Sons, Inc., New York, 1971.

Drucker, Peter F.: *The Effective Executive*, Harper and Row, New York, 1967.

Essert, Paul L.: *Creative Leadership in Adult Education*, Prentice-Hall, New York, 1951.

Hallenbeck, Wilbur C.: "Reflections of an Adult Educator," *Adult Educ.*, **16**(3): 169-174, 1966.

Hassenplug, Lulu W.: "The Good Teacher," *Nurs. Outlook*, **13**(10): 24-27, 1965.

Houle, Cyril O.: "The Education of Edult Educational Leaders," *Handbook of Adult Education in the United States*, Adult Education Association of the U.S.A., Chicago, 1960, Chap. 10, pp. 117-128.

_____: "The Educators of Adults," *Handbook of Adult Education*, The Macmillan Company, New York, 1970, Chap. 7, pp. 109-119.

Knowles, Malcolm S.: *Informal Adult Education: A Guide for Administrators, Leaders, and Teachers*, Association Press, New York, 1950.

Kramer, Marlene: "Does Teacher Really Know Best?" *J. Nurs. Educ.*, **6**(1): 3-11; 24-27, 1967.

Liveright, A. A.: *Strategies of Leadership in Conducting Adult Education Programs*, Harper and Brothers, New York, 1959.

Merton, Robert K.: "The Nature of Leadership," *Int. Nurs. Rev.*, **16**(4): 310-319, 1969.

Miller, Harry L.: *Teaching and Learning in Adult Education*, Macmillan Company, New York, 1964.

Nahm, Helen: "Faculty Responsibility," *Nurs. Forum*, **1**(4): 14-17, 1962.

Osborn, Alex F.: *Applied Imagination*, 3d ed., Charles Scribner's Sons, New York, 1963.

Peterson, Houston (ed.): *Great Teachers Portrayed By Those Who Studied Under Them*, Vantage Books, New York, 1946.

Popiel, Elda: "The Director of Continuing Education in Perspective," *Nurs. Forum*, **8**(1): 86-93, 1969.

Rogers, Carl: *Freedom to Learn*, Charles E. Merrill Publishing Company, Columbus, Ohio, 1969.

Schlotfeldt, Rozella M.: "Nursing in the University Community," *Nurs. Forum*, **5**(1): 22-27, 1966.

Schweer, Jean E.: "Continuing Education Climatology," *J. Nurs. Adm.*, **1**(1): 45-48, 1971.

_____: *Creative Teaching in Clinical Nursing*, 2d ed. The C. V. Mosby Company, St. Louis, 1972.

8

Methods of teaching

The nurse who performs nursing procedures by rote rather than by reason is an anachronism today. And so is the teacher in continuing nursing education whose teaching is based solely on precedence and personal expedience.

The previous chapter points out the many desirable characteristics of the teacher and the administrator in continuing nursing education. This chapter which deals with methods and modes of instruction further substantiates the need for those characteristics.

After the philosophical and theoretical framework of the curriculum are established and objectives developed and accepted, decisions are made concerning appropriate content and methods to be used in reaching the objectives. Whether the content is viewed as important in itself or as a means to an end depends on the learning theory held; however, content is necessary in any event to provide a focus for learning. Mechanisms to be used in the teaching-learning transaction are selected on the basis of their best potential to fulfill the learning mission.

TYPES OF METHODS

Consideration of the content and the means by which learning will take place proceeds from the level of generalization to progressively more specific levels. Teaching strategies may be viewed as being at the level of generalization. If principles of adult education are accepted as generalizations, they may be regarded as teaching strategies. For example, one principle is "start where the learner is in terms of his readiness to learn." To adopt the principle as a strategy means that a decision is made to base the teaching-learning process on the learner's experience and knowledge. But that strategy does not tell us the methods which will carry out its accomplishment.

Methods are based on curriculum planning decisions made in accordance with adopted strategies and appropriate to the sponsoring institution or agency. To continue with the example given in the preceding paragraph, one method to implement the strategy is to establish that "an assessment of entry level knowledge, and behavior of the learner will be conducted as an essential part of the program." Again, that method does not tell us which techniques, procedures, or devices are to be used in carrying out the assessment.

The decision determining the specific techniques, procedures, or devices to be used lies within the province of the particular faculty member responsible for the actual teaching. Obviously a variety of ways exists to gain evidence of assessments such as checklists, questionnaires, essays, discussions, or interviews, to name only a few. In some instances an additional device such as a filmed, videotaped, or audiotaped sequence may be used as an integral part of the technique which the teacher uses. The prerecorded sequence may be used to establish a situation as the focal point for an essay.

Methods then are not always specific in identifying precise techniques or tools to be used in teaching but they do provide a framework or guide for the nurse teacher as established for the curriculum in which he is involved. At this point a discussion of types of methods may be useful. The three types which follow are developed from the learner's point of view.

Dependent Methods

Nurses are especially aware of the hazards of labeling or categorizing anything; yet, for purposes of discussion, even an arbitrary typing of methods may help to sort out different ways of approaching the teaching-learning transaction. Dependent methods are those in which the learner exerts little control or influence on how the information is incorporated into class activities. In other words the learner is expected to rely on administrative or teaching decisions to determine what information is to be provided, when, how much, where, and in what manner.

The communication pathway in a dependent method is often limited to a one-way direction from teacher to learner. Thus lectures, demonstrations, and other formal presentations are examples of dependent methods. In a nation which values independence and in a profession which holds the same value, dependency seems to have negative connotations. However, dependent methods are far from deserving a completely negative rating.

Despite disadvantages of a one-way flow of communication, methods such as the formal lecture or demonstration may be the most efficient way in a given situation to achieve a selected objective. When content or subject matter is to be communicated to a group of learners in a short time, a dependent method may be chosen for reasons of space, time, and economy.

In continuing nursing education, the next learning methods are growing in favor among some learners. Self-directed learning and independent study are terms which are becoming increasingly familiar.

Independent Methods

When the learner is able to control the pacing for his learning, the subject matter, the place, time, or length of study, an independent method is in use. From the learner's point of view the teaching-learning environment is such that he may select and engage in the learning activities of his choice to meet his learning objectives.

Independent methods include a number of techniques and devices such as programmed instruction, computer-assisted instruction, and retrieval systems as described in Chapter 12. The multimedia learning carrels discussed in Chapter 13 are also means to carry through independent methods for learning.

In contrasting dependent and independent methods, the latter is likely to benefit from a halo effect which may not be deserved. Independent methods are often thought of as being innovative, creative, or learner-centered, more so than dependent methods. The hazard is that if each method is the only method, no choice of methods exists. Since individuals learn in their own unique ways, a choice of methods is as important as choices within a method.

One of the ways to sustain interest in learning and at the same time add to the choices of learning experiences is to consider the teaching-learning milieu. The teacher, the learner, and the group comprise a force which may be useful to an educational effort.

Interdependent Methods

The flow of communication and control of learning experiences are shared between teacher and learner and among learners in interdependent methods of learning. Each member of the group carries individual responsibility for participating and directing learning for himself and carries some measure of the collective responsibility for the group's learning.

Interdependent methods are characterized by the group participants working together, discussing, exploring, questioning, and testing out aspects of the learning process which concern the group as a whole. When the learner is a part of a group, his pace of progress in learning is influenced by other members of the group. At the same time, he is influencing the pace or progress in learning among group members. Thus interdependence is operational within the group.

Parts of informational content being used or extended through interdependent methods are obtained in various ways including dependent and independent methods as well as interdependent methods. Seldom will a sponsoring agency be so restrictive as to limit itself to one type of method, regardless of the flexibility of techniques available within it.

A brief review of the three methods recounted here will reveal that each of them may incorporate and use to advantage selected instructional materials and approaches. For example, a motion picture with or without sound is apt to add a dimension to any one of the three methods equally well.

SELECTED INSTRUCTIONAL APPROACHES

Words such as *educational media* usually bring to mind filmed or televised content. The words commonly imply the use of an electrical or electronic device. Familiar and time-tested vehicles of communication such as printed words are mistakenly regarded as traditional tools rather than as the rightful educational media which they are. Thus the title for this section of the chapter uses *instructional approaches* as a broadly encompassing term which includes more than technological means. The term *selected* appears in the section title because both a detailed survey and comprehensive discussion of materials and approaches are beyond the scope of this chapter. Yet the application or use of some concepts and developments in various educational efforts are appropriate and may be of interest as related to continuing nursing education. The references cited for this chapter are useful as guides to a more inclusive consideration of various approaches which are only briefly dealt with or omitted in this discussion. Furthermore, where local resources include educational specialists with expertise in the development and use of particular approaches, consultation may be advantageous.

Simulation

Adults have learned the usefulness of the let's pretend approach either when they were children or as they worked with children. The landings on the moon as reported by the national television networks demonstrated the value of simulations in the aerospace training program and for reporting. Given some background information and structure as a frame of reference, the human imagination is capable of stimulating responses in a lifelike situation which are valid indicators of responses to a real life situation.

In nursing, simulation in some forms is quite familiar. The Mary Chase mannikin, the old nursing arts' classroom which replicated a hospital unit, and even a colleague as a pretend patient are all ready examples of simulation. Talking with professional nurses who took their state board nursing examinations in the 1930s reveals that in many instances a practical part was included in the testing using a simulated situation in which the candidate was expected to perform an assignment as in actual patient care.

Simulated situations are useful means to gain learner involvement and group interaction, to provide practice in problem solving and decision making, and to elicit demonstrations of behavior. Because situations may be adapted to a familiar or meaningful context for the learner, simulation offers ways of learning and practicing the learnings in the safe setting of the classroom. A quick and obvious example in nursing is the use of the mannikin for learning external cardiac massage and mouth to mouth resuscitation. The opportunity to learn to cope effectively in an emergency situation is provided, combining theory, application of theory, practice, feedback, and reinforcement of learning and evaluation as the nurse performs with a simulated cardiac arrest patient. Emergencies as a concept are familiar and meaningful to nurses. Their motivations to learn about a specific emergency may be heightened if practice is offered even in a simulated situation rather than merely being presented with the content.

Perhaps because life is seldom static, the use of simulated life events connotes some action. In today's fast-moving culture, action seems to have value for at least a segment of nurse learners who enjoy learning through participative methods. The following discussion provides a few examples of simulation techniques as components of interdependent methods of teaching.

Role Playing. As a teaching-learning form, role playing is particularly useful for developing communication skills, involving emotions, and encouraging group work. Different from a prepared skit, play, playlet, or a dramatized presentation where a cast of characters follow scripts written in advance of presentation, role playing depends upon the spontaneity of the participants. Role playing also differs from the psychodrama since psychodrama focuses on the private problems of the person, while role playing focuses on common problems among individuals sharing a social role such as that of the nurse. The realistic degree to which the role players are able to enact a situation may well be a reflection of the understanding, insight, and involvement of the learners and the relevance that the simulated event has for the participants.

The teacher in continuing nursing education who includes role playing in course work may use the technique as a result of class discussion. For example, in a discussion of supervisory problems in nursing, several nurse learners may wish the class to consider approaches in working with a member of the nursing staff who is consistently tardy. One particular instance may be selected by the group as a representative case and further information about that situation may be sought.

After class members are acquainted with the description of the situation and the persons involved, volunteers to role play are solicited. Because of personal inhibitions among class members and because they are adults meriting adult treatment, role players are selected on a voluntary basis rather than assignment. If more than one teacher is available, role playing by the instructional staff provides an opportunity for the class members to observe an operational demonstration of the technique. Such observation may be an effective way of encouraging participation.

As role playing is an interdependent method of teaching, maintaining the voluntary aspect in assuming the roles is important. Admittedly, if the concept of role playing is totally new to everyone in the class and if the class members have not yet developed some common feelings for one another, they may not wish to engage in it until a later time when familiarity has developed. The teacher respects the group's decision which then calls for a different technique, such as open discussion, to be used.

When volunteers are obtained for the roles, they are advised to enact their roles according to the information elicited from the previous discussion. The instructor may wish to label each player with a card designating the role being taken and to caution them against stepping outside of their roles at any time during the role playing sequence. The volunteers proceed with the enactment of a simulated situation without benefit of any coaching or rehearsal as soon as the observers have been reminded that the purpose here is to consider, analyze, and assess effective approaches in working with the consistently tardy staff member.

The length of time that one role playing sequence should take is comparable to the correct dosage of any medication; it should be enough. Too little or too much will detract from its impact. When the observing group has noted the direction and substance of the content enough to enable analysis of the approach or the players to arrive at closure, the sequence is ended.

A brief and to the point process to de-role the players takes place immediately following the sequence and before any discussion is permitted. The teacher may accomplish de-rolement in several ways such as calling the players by their own names rather than the names assumed for their roles, shaking their hands, or asking the observers to applaud the work of the volunteers. Applause by action and sound interrupts the simulation and vividly recalls the entire group to reality. To further assure de-rolement, the teacher may give the players the first opportunity to comment on or analyze the roles portrayed.

Any discussion which ensues from role playing focuses objectively on the determinants of the process to gain information and to use constructive approaches—in this instance, in working with the person who is consistently tardy. The analysis takes place within the framework of the problem for which a solution is sought and not with regard to the quality of acting. Facts or information given, behavior observed, and statements made in the role playing sequence are the basis for the analysis. The observers are so called because discussion is intended to stem from observations, not opinions.

As a consequence of thoughtful discussion, the teacher may assist the class in either developing suggested actions for the future or arriving at some general guidelines which might be useful as reference for similar or related situations. If the class is inclined to test out the findings of its analysis, the teacher may suggest another sequence of role playing which incorporates the actions or guidelines developed. Whether the same or different volunteers are involved in the second sequence is immaterial and optional as the focus is on process and not on specific persons.

Other ways to provide practice or reinforcement of learning from the role-playing and discussion activities are available. One way is a variant of role playing which may involve the total class through writing. A situation is described and each class member is to assume a common role, such as the role of the nurse, in the situation. Each member then responds in writing, stating the actions, reasons, and thoughts he incorporates into his role playing.

Recognizing that some individuals are more comfortable than others in expressing their thoughts in writing, written work may generate different responses. Discussion is based on the written responses which are regarded as anonymous contributions. Tabulation of responses may be enlightening to teacher and learners alike and may well stimulate further discussion, reading, and examination of issues.

Dramatized Presentations. Occasionally, a play is a technique which may be used to either provide content, set a mood, or review the ramifications of a problem. If experienced actors are available, the dramatization is likely to be more realistic than if amateurs participate. When learners are free to concentrate on the play's message rather than be distracted by the quality of role enactment, the objective for using the play may better be satisfied.

Because the human imagination is capable of filling in a number of gaps that may exist, perfect simulation is not a prerequisite. For example, if the play calls for a telephone, a telephone does not actually have to be obtained and used, or a table may be used instead of a desk.

Dramatized presentations require advanced planning and coordination with a number of individuals but, if well done, are a productive and different approach. Another way to provide a format for learning through involvement and activity is by use of simulation games.

Simulation Games. A sense of fun and frivolity is often associated with games. Competition and endurance may also be associated. In a more serious vein, life's hurdles may be likened to the hurdles in a game. Although games are not new as devices used in teaching, either simple games or games depending on a simulated environment have not been widely used in continuing nursing education. In the past some people used to think that unless medicine had a bad taste, its efficacy was questionable. Are there some nursing educators who fear that unless the teaching methods are conventional, the effectiveness of learning will suffer? Are there others who believe that games are more appropriate to children and youth than to adults and professionals?

An increasing interest in the value of simulation games is found among social scientists, management and business trainers, and teachers of general adult education. While further research is needed to assess the impact on learning, games appear to have positive and productive effects at least for some learners. Since each of us learns best in different ways, one can hardly expect unanimity in responses. Yet experience indicates that the value of simulation games as a teaching tool may not yet be appreciated fully.

In the simulation of a life situation for a game, care is taken to build in and reflect reality factors. The nurse educator who wishes to invent and develop a game as a means to meet a particular learning objective may well use anonymous actual clinical data as needed to reflect reality.

A story is told of an invisible herd of forty cows which provides students with experience in dairy herd breeding and management. The bovines exist only on computer tape, allowing students to simulate twenty years of scientific breeding in a matter of weeks. Individual or group management of the cows is presumably possible. Thus the management of the herd may be seen as a variant form of a simulation game.

Just as solitaire is a game of cards for one individual, simulation games may be for one person. But games may involve either sole or multiple players. Because the objective for such games is educational rather than diversional, winning is not a constant criterion of success. The *in-basket exercise,* described in detail in a handbook published by the Hospital Research and Educational Trust, provides a good example of a simulation technique that does not depend on winning or losing the game.[1] Individuals compare and contrast their performance with other members of the class in accordance with the instructional goals.

Success is regarded in different forms according to the purpose of the game. For example, if the purpose of a game is to provide practice in verbal and nonverbal communication skills in planning and carrying out a group assignment, the criteria for success may include the group's participative behavior and the verbalized feelings of accomplishment, satisfaction, and learning as a result of the game even when the group does not win. Other advantages of group games include those aspects which are conducive to the participation of the quiet members of a class and to the encouragement given by the situation for nurses to learn from each other as playing proceeds.

Of the relatively few games which have been developed thus far, none is directly concerned with nursing practice but some may be useful with minimal or no adaptation to continuing nursing education. For example, a simulation game which was developed for an aspect of supervision in business and industry may be useful for that same aspect in a continuing nursing education course on supervision.

Ideally, simulation games are researched and developed with care, using theoretical constructs from which basic principles may be operationalized. Thus the teacher who intends to use or adapt a specific game is cautioned to become acquainted with those research findings if they are available before a firm decision to adopt or adapt the game is made. Furthermore, such findings may provide a guide for modification. Boocock and Schild have included a listing of centers involved in gaming research and development.[2]

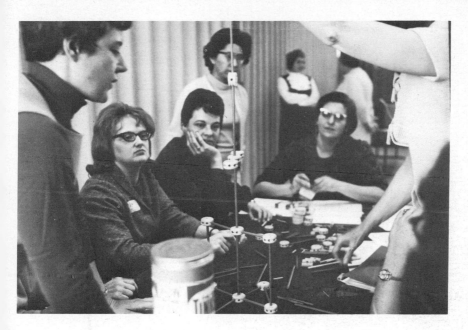

Figure 8-1   Familiar equipment in a simulation game.

As is true in using any other method of teaching, the physical environment of the learners is planned to be appropriate for the activities involved. Usually a room with movable rather than fixed seats is desirable. Tables rather than chairs with arm desks may be required. Adequate floor space for prescribed activities may be necessary. If a variety of supplies and equipment is used, all will need to be ready and on hand. Useful materials may be very familiar or completely strange (see Fig. 8-1). In addition the instructor may wish to suggest to the class that a particular form of dress—pant suits or slacks—is recommended for the gaming session's activities.

Whether role playing, simulation games, or other provocative modes of instruction such as the incident process and case method are adopted by continuing nursing educators, awareness of commonalities among the methods is helpful. Pigors and his colleagues make the point that both the incident process and the case situation are based solidly on past or present realities of a true circumstance.[3] True-to-life depiction and reporting may be accomplished in several ways, but beyond the details of authenticity lies the common denominator, a need for follow-up activities with all instructional approaches.

Follow-up activities include provision of feedback to learner and teacher through planned efforts such as group discussions, written exercises, or debates. Analytic problem solving may be practiced with guidance so that nurse learners become skilled in assessing and constructively considering, if not always resolving, identified questions. Follow-up activities usually include some aspects of evaluation to guide learning. Without dwelling further on the obvious need for follow-up activities, the next discussion will consider another innovation in simulated approaches.

Trigger Films. The concept underlying the production and use of trigger films is not new to continuing nursing education. When Mary Hill was director of continuing education in nursing at the University of Pittsburgh, she developed and used short realistic situations recorded on videotape to elicit response and discussion in classes regarding the clinical care of patients. More recently trigger films, as one- to three-minute simulations of particular situations, are being developed at the University of Michigan in content areas as diverse as driver or drug education, gerontology, and mental retardation.[4]

Each film focuses on a central theme and is designed to establish a certain evocative situation. The film is stopped at a point appropriate for discussion by the target audience. A final close-up of an emotional facial expression or a challenging question such as "What would you do?" at the end of the film may stimulate consideration of an analysis of situations like those portrayed in the films.

An added variation to the use of the trigger film is being developed in an extension consumer education program at the University of Wisconsin.[5] After completion of discussion, the film is continued with the characters stepping outside of their roles and explaining what they were doing in the film.

Study guides for learners and discussion guides for teachers are helpful for proper use of trigger films. While no specific formula, sequence, or format exists for producing such films, general criteria require that the mission to be accomplished by any particular film be very specific and unified. Terms such as *single-concept films* have tended to be misused and adapted to certain forms of film loops rather than used to acknowledge one conceptual focus. A trigger film is a single-concept film in an authentic way and considers one clear purpose, one succinct situation, and an identifiable mood and direction.

Other Simulation Methods. In the transitional period between radio and television, phonograph records and audiotapes gained recognition as aids in teaching. Although the visual dimension was limited to the mind's eye, audio presentations of nurse-patient interactions were simulated for educational purposes and were and are useful today. However, with the advances in technology and the growing expectation of materials which provide both sight and sound, videotapes, slides and audiotape combinations, and other resources are increasingly available. With the advent of cassettes and cartridges associated with motion picture projectors and television monitors, the mobility of equipment

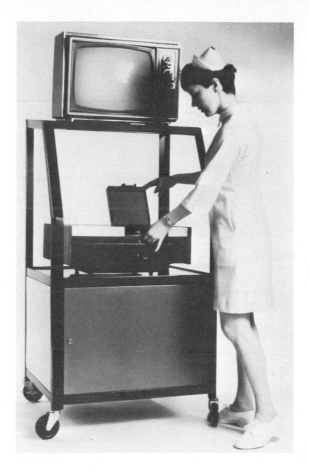

Figure 8-2 Cassette player and standard television
set. (*Motorola Systems Inc., Chicago*)

and ease of viewing has been enhanced. Electronically videorecorded film is
capable of playback from a player on any standard television set (see Fig. 8-2).
Disk recording of television content is also under research and development.
Multiple means are found for the instructor who wishes to employ simulation
techniques in continuing education courses in nursing.

Special Telephone/Radio Networks

Although the telephone and radio are two distinct media, they may be
used in combination to provide the learner with a choice in the method he will

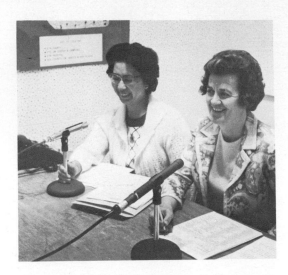

Figure 8-3   Speaker and moderator in a sound studio, the point of
origin for a telephone/radio network class.

use to participate in coursework. When used in combination, the message is
carried from the point of origin simultaneously on the telephone and radio to
the listening audience (see Fig. 8-3). With a telephone network, the learner may
communicate directly to others on the line from the network phone at his
listening post. With the radio, unless a two-way system is in effect, the learner
needs to use a regular telephone, place a long distance call to the point of class
origin, and ask to speak to the instructor instead of being instantly in direct
communication.

A telephone or radio network established for educational purposes involves either telephones with voice amplifiers which are connected to private
lines contracted to form the system, or radios which are capable of receiving the
band being used. As an instructional approach which enables contact with nurses
from a variety of geographic and occupational locations, the number of networks in the nation have increased from one in 1957 to many more today.
States with networks include for example Minnesota, Nebraska, New York,
Ohio, West Virginia, and Wisconsin.

Because the telephone and radio are audio media, visual supplements
require deliberate and careful planning. An outline of key points for a tele-
phone/radio class is useful to the learner and serves as a means of clarifying and
reinforcing learning. If slides are used, multiple sets need to be developed and
distributed, one set to each listening post. Every post will also require a slide

projector, a screen, and at least one person who is familiar with the operation of the equipment. Where possible, information given on slides is repeated with the outline of the lecture to assure good visibility and adequate time for viewing. Such repeated information also has value for the learner who wishes to review the material later and to study independently.

A few suggested references for independent and more detailed study at the end of a class outline may be helpful if the learner has some access to the references. The inclusion of reprints in a course syllabus may be particularly appreciated by nurses whose library resources locally are severely limited.

Suggestions for activities before and after the class may encourage the learner to become involved in preparation for and as follow-up to the class. Where a local discussion follows the telephone/radio class the relationship and application of the lecture content to local practice and concerns may be explored. However the degree to which local discussions may reinforce or extend the class content undoubtedly depends on the nursing leadership available in the setting.

For example, if a case study is to be the focus of a particular class, prepared materials which include the salient case study information and specific references as a reading assignment may be mailed to learners in advance of the class time. A nurse leader in concert with other nurses at a given listening post may be able to relate certain aspects about the case study subject's clinical situation to a parallel or similar one familiar to the nurses in that setting. Where complete differences exist, an analysis to explain the variations may be a productive topic of discussion to follow the telephone/radio class.

The potential for outreach implicit in the use of the telephone/radio approach cannot be negated. But, as with all approaches involving mass media, instructional benefits may vary according to the congruency, consistency, and control which can be integrated into the curriculum. For example, classes intended for registered nurses may build upon basic content which they may be assumed to have. Yet, if control of learners' attendance at listening posts is not possible and nursing assistants or licensed practical nurses attend classes intended for registered nurses, the learning outcomes may not be congruent or consistent with the planned program. Reaching particular target learners is an issue which has not been entirely resolved.

Teaching-Learning Assignments

Other approaches which may merit consideration in continuing nursing education are adaptations of activities which may not be new to the nurse as a learner or a practitioner. Because most of the learners involved in continuing nursing education are practicing nurses, the curriculum sequence is often planned to allow for developmental or application phases. For example, a course may be planned to meet for a total of three weeks over a two-month period. According to the time available in the practice setting, assignments relating to course content may be not only appropriate but also desirable as a planned instructional approach to assure better synthesis of learning.

Case study, nursing care planning, process recording, patient assessment, and documenting observations are possibilities, to name only a few activities which may be used as assignments to enhance learning and to reinforce the relevance of content to practice. When such assignments are used discussion and feedback to the learner are considered essential but may be on an individual or group basis. Flexibility and room for the learner to pursue a project of personal interest or relevance are important in the consideration of assignments.

Nurse-patient interviews as well as talks or demonstrations by patients are also useful approaches to instruction. Involvement of patients certainly tends to heighten the validity of continuing nursing education content for some learners and may be the key to involvement for others. To read about the patient in generalities in a textbook is far different from hearing the experiences or perceptions of an identifiable person. As nurses learn to care for and work with the person and his family, nurses may become more comfortable with the notion that just as teaching and learning are reciprocal concepts, so are nurses and patients reciprocals as teaching-learning takes place.

The seminar approach in continuing nursing education is especially useful. A group of learners, with guidance and supervision from the educator, study and discuss subjects of mutual concern. Preclass assignments are likely to arise from the group members as the group explores and progresses in its learning activities. Any formal presentations may be an outcome of a particular aspect studied by one or more of the class members. Because the seminar approach assumes some basic knowledge and understandings, the method is helpful for peer groups in promoting involvement and participation.

The following chapter will serve to delineate further considerations in the conduct and presentation of continuing nursing education offerings.

Notes

1. *Training and Continuing Education: A Handbook for Health Care Institutions,* Hospital Research and Educational Trust, Chicago, 1970, pp. 168-175.

2. Sarane S. Boocock, and E. O. Schild (eds.), *Simulation Games in Learning,* Sage Publications, Inc., Beverly Hills, California, 1968, pp. 275-279.

3. Paul Pigors, Faith Pigors, and Marita Tribo, *Professional Nursing Practice: Cases and Issues,* McGraw-Hill Book Company, New York, 1967, p. 6.

4. Ellen J. Miller, "Trigger Filmmaking," *Audiovisual Instruction,* 16(5): 64-67 1971.

5. "Consumer Program Uses Trigger Film," *University Extension News the University of Wisconsin,* 8, 5(2): 1972.

REFERENCES

Bergevin, Paul, John McKinley, and Robert M. Smith: "The Adult Education Activity: Content, Processes, and Procedures," in G. Jensen, A. A. Liveright, and W. Hallenbeck (eds.), *Adult Education Outlines of an Emerging Field of University Study*, Adult Education Association of the U.S.A., 1964, Chap. 14, pp. 270-289.

Boocock, Sarane S., and E. O. Schild (eds.): *Simulation Games in Learning*, Sage Publications, Inc., Beverly Hills, California, 1968.

Brown, James W. and Kenneth Norberg: *Administering Educational Media*, McGraw-Hill Book Company, New York, 1965.

Brunner, Edmund deS., David S. Wilder, Corinne Kirchner, and John S. Newberry, Jr.: *An Overview of Adult Education Research*, Adult Education Association of the U.S.A., Chicago, 1959.

Cabeceiras, James: "Systematizing a Nursing Degree Program 'ILL' " *Audiovisual Instruction*, 16(10): 12-15, 1971.

Calvert, Donald E.: "Management Games as Teaching Devices," *Training and Development Journal*, 24(2): 16-18, 1970.

"Consumer Program Uses Trigger Film," *University Extension News The University of Wisconsin*, 5(2): 8, 1972.

Craig, Robert L., and Lester R. Bittel, eds.: *Training and Development Handbook*, McGraw-Hill Book Company, New York, 1967.

de Tornyay, Rheba: *Strategies for Teaching Nursing*, John Wiley and Sons, Inc., New York, 1971.

Hamilton, Carl H.: "University Learning Resources and Instructional Management," *Educational Technology*, 11(5): 14-16, 1971.

Heidgerken, Loretta E.: *Teaching and Learning in Schools of Nursing Principles and Methods*, 3d ed., J. B. Lippincott Company, Philadelphia, 1965.

Hornback, May S.: "University Sponsored Staff Education in Nursing via a Telephone/Radio Network," *Int. J. Nurs. Stud.*, 6(4): 217-223, 1969.

How To Use Role Playing and Other Tools for Learning, Leadership Pamphlet No. 6, Adult Education Association of the U.S.A., Chicago, 1956.

Kemp, Jerold E.: *Instructional Design: A Plan for Unit and Course Development*, Fearon Publishers, Belmont, California, 1971.

Kidd, J. R.: *How Adults Learn*, Association Press, New York, 1959, pp. 232-269.

Knowles, Malcolm S.: *The Modern Practice of Adult Education*, Association Press, New York, 1970, pp. 292-297.

Lange, Phil C. (ed.): *Programmed Instruction: The Sixty-sixth Yearbook of the National Society for the Study of Education Part II*, The University of Chicago Press, Chicago, 1967.

MacDonald, James B.: "Strategies of Instruction in Adult Education," *Adult Learning and Instruction*, Stanley M. Grabowski (ed.), ERIC Clearinghouse on Adult Education and Adult Education Association of the U.S.A., Syracuse, New York, 1970.

Miller, Ellen J.: "Trigger Filmmaking," *Audiovisual Instruction*, 16(5): 64-67, 1971.

Niles, Anne McKee: "Call 'Nursing Dial Access' " *Amer. J. Nurs.*, 69(6): 1235-1236, 1969.

Peterson, Carol J.: "Multi-Sensory Tutorial Instruction in Associate Degree Nursing Education," *Audiovisual Instruction*, 16(10): 16-18, 1971.

Pigors, Paul, Faith Pigors, and Marita Tribo: *Professional Nursing Practice: Cases and Issues*, McGraw-Hill Book Company, New York, 1967.

Puzzeroli, David A., and Charles J. Fazzaro: *The Development of Telelecture and Associated Media Systems for the Improvement of Nursing Education in West Virginia*, West Virginia University, Morgantown, August 1971.

Redman, Barbara K., and Shirley J. Harlow: "Instructional Qualities of Television Visuals for Fundamentals of Nursing," *J. Nurs. Educ.*, 35-41, 8(4): 1969.

Skinner, B. F.: *The Technology of Teaching*, Meredith Corporation, New York, 1968.

Tough, Allen M.: *Learning Without a Teacher—A Study of Tasks and Assistance During Adult Self-Teaching Projects*, The Ontario Institute for Studies in Education, Ontario, 1967.

Training and Continuing Education: A Handbook for Health Care Institutions, Hospital Research and Educational Trust, Chicago, 1970.

Warren, Virginia B., ed.: "Simulation Techniques: How and Why," *Techniques for Teachers of Adults*, 12(4): 1-4, 1972.

————: *The Second Treasury of Techniques for Teaching Adults*, National Association for Public Continuing and Adult Education, Washington, D.C., 1970.

Weidenbach, Ernestine: *Meeting the Realities in Clinical Teaching*, Springer Publishing Company, Inc., New York, 1969.

Wolf, Vivian C.: "Some Implications of Short-Term, Long-Term Memory Theory," *Nurs. Forum*, 150-165, 10(2): 1971.

9

Conferences, workshops, institutes, and clinical courses

The short-term course is a popular format for educational offerings designed for practicing nurses. Such a course provides the opportunity for nurses to leave the employment setting for short periods of time, thus permitting some educational endeavor for those unable to enroll in full-time educational pursuits.

Short-term courses often have a workshop, conference, or institute format. Many of the principles relating to planning and conducting these sessions are similar so are considered together in this chapter.

There are some distinctions between each of these types of meetings, although in common usage the terms are often used interchangeably. *Clinical courses* involve a combination of the elements of each but concentrate on planned, supervised clinical experience. Clinical courses bear a strong resemblance to the older postgraduate nursing courses (discussed in Chapter 2) but are more soundly planned, and are based on the needs of the learners.

Workshops, conferences, and institutes are defined in Chapter 1. To review, an *institute* is usually seen as a series of lectures, often by different speakers, with a minimum of audience participation. The institute is suitable for transmitting knowledge and relating experience, but the extent of the learning gained by passive sitting and listening is questionable, particularly when the sessions extend over long periods of time. Because of the heavy reliance on the lecture method of teaching, institutes are usually of short duration, from one to three days. The effectiveness of an institute depends upon the skill of the teacher in involving the audience in the presentation and in his ability to inspire participants to act upon the information presented.

Conferences and *workshops* are more informal approaches to education.

135

The conference is probably the most frequently used approach to continuing education in nursing for it emphasizes group problem-solving. Someone has said that "for finding the right answer, the conference can be the best thing since the back of your arithmetic book!" That statement may be a bit over-enthusiastic, but it reflects the adaptability of the conference for many different purposes and groups.

The *conference* permits a pooling of various points of view and a sharing of experiences that lead to joint thinking. It requires a skillful leader, but it depends heavily upon audience participation, and requires that participants contribute from their own knowledge and experience. Demonstrations, talks, role playing, learning games, films and other audiovisual media may all be used as a basis for conference participation.

Workshops are also planned to involve the participants in specific tasks related to the subject. The workshop is characterized by audience involvement and is usually designed for experienced persons to study problems of mutual concern. Working subgroups are organized around interest areas in task-oriented or problem-solving situations. As its name implies, the workshop requires work, and the results of that work may be in the concrete form of recommendations, reports, or specific tools. Institutional workshops are appropriate for certain types of activities, such as designing nursing care plans or other patient care tools, or in instituting changes, such as the nursing audit.

PLANNING

The number of meetings planned for nurses by various groups is constantly increasing. This is obviously in response to an expression of learning needs, for without feeling the need, nurses would not usually attend. Yet considerable time, effort, and money are expended, both by the individual and usually by the employing agency as well. Therefore any offering should be carefully planned and executed.

Without adequate planning it is difficult to avoid duplication of efforts. In determining content, faculty of educational institutions should not design programs that might be done more effectively by another group, such as a nursing organization. The reverse is also true.

The elements of planning are presented in Chapter 6. These principles of planning apply to any type of educational endeavor, so will not be repeated in detail here, but the reader may find it useful to refer to that chapter.

Some of the details of planning for short-term courses may be a little different than for other types of educational pursuits. To assist the planner, a workshop planning guide is presented in Exhibit 9.1.

Exhibit 9.1   WORKSHOP PLANNING GUIDE

Purposes and Objectives

1. Have the purposes of the workshop been clearly defined?
2. Is there evidence of need for the workshop?
3. Are the objectives clearly stated?
4. Are the objectives stated in measurable terms?
5. Are criteria or prerequisites clearly stated?
6. Have enrollment limitations been defined?

Content and Presentation

7. Is the designated content appropriate to meeting the objectives?
8. Is the length of time for the workshop adequate for meeting the objectives?
9. Have suitable teaching methods been selected?
10. Have appropriate teaching faculty been selected?
11. Have discussion leaders, recorders, and resource people been appointed?
12. Have all faculty and staff participants been adequately oriented?
13. Are useful audiovisual aids and other teaching materials available or can they be developed?
14. Is preparation or advance study required of participants? Have necessary materials been mailed to them?

Budget and Finance

15. Is the workshop adequately budgeted?
16. Have fees been established?
17. Are obligations of sponsors and co-sponsors clearly defined?

Equipment and Facilities

18. Is necessary equipment available or must it be borrowed?
19. Are suitable facilities available?

(continued)

Exhibit 9.1 CONTINUED

20. Are room arrangements suitable for the teaching methods selected?
21. Are adequate housing arrangements located nearby?
22. Have arrangements for meals been made?
23. Is parking space available?
24. Has hospitality been provided for?
25. Are arrangements for recreation necessary?

Promotion and Publicity

26. Have promotional materials been developed?
27. Do promotional materials stimulate interest and explain the workshop clearly?
28. Is there an adequate mailing list for direct mailings?
29. Has radio, television, and newspaper publicity been provided for?
30. Have adequate arrangements been made for enrollment and registration?

Evaluation

31. Have evaluation tools been developed?
32. Are plans being made for any follow-up of the workshop?

Selection of appropriate physical facilities is also a responsibility of course planners. A check list for these facilities is given in Exhibit 9.2. More information on arrangements about these facilities may be found in Chapter 13.

PURPOSES AND OBJECTIVES

The purpose of the educational activity should be very clear to the planners and should be expressed in such a way that it is also clear to potential enrollees. This statement is identified in the descriptive flier to help the prospective enrollees determine the usefulness of the activity to them.

Purposes of short-term educational pursuits may vary. Often the purpose is *the presentation of new information*; an added purpose is to attempt *to motivate* the participants to change nursing practice by the application of knowledge gained. Other courses may be designed as *skill-training* sessions.

Exhibit 9.2   FACILITIES CHECKLIST

(A facilities checklist is a guide for conference planning.)

	Available	Not required		Available	Not required
Coat room			Visual aids		
Registration area			bulletin board		
chairs			chalkboard		
conference			chalk and		
materials			eraser		
name tags			flannel board		
tables			flip chart		
Conference room			extra		
ash trays			newsprint		
chairs and			felt pens		
tables			Projectors		
drinking water			8 mm		
and glasses			16 mm		
exhibit space			slide		
lectern			opaque		
lighting			overhead		
name cards			Screen		
and holders			Tape recorder		
notepads			blank tapes		
paper and			TV monitor		
pencils			Other:		
question cards					
sound system					
storage space					
other					

Another purpose may be *to provide inspiration* to enrollees. *Exchange of experiences* is another important purpose for conferences and workshops, although these sessions may also provide opportunities for *problem solving.* In certain kinds of learning experiences, a *commitment to action* by participants is an expected outcome.

Whatever the purpose, it should be clearly defined. Confusion or disagreement between the faculty and the participants over purposes is not only disrupting, it is unfair to those attending.

Determining Objectives

Effective conduct of any educational offering requires a specific determination of its objectives, and the short term course is no exception. These objectives should be spelled out in as much detail as possible. (It may be helpful to refer to the example in Exhibit 6.3).

To identify specific objectives, course planners must have a clear understanding of what is to be accomplished. Participants must also have this understanding; ideally the objectives are worked out by planners and participants and are mutually acceptable. Otherwise, flexible planning permits an alteration of the stated objectives if participants find them unacceptable.

Secondary purposes or objectives, sometimes identified as the hidden agenda, are rarely defined in establishing objectives for programs, but planning is more effective if these objectives are understood. They include such goals as renewing former acquaintances, meeting new people, revitalizing a feeling of belonging to a group, or broadening one's viewpoint. Secondary objectives may be primary for some participants; for example, a nurse attending the conference may not be primarily interested in the content, but wants to get away from the job for a few days or to have the opportunity to go shopping in the city where the course is being held. If these secondary goals take precedence over the course objectives, faculty will encounter difficulty in conducting the course.

Consideration of secondary objectives means allowing a certain amount of free time, adequate time for coffee breaks, and, in long programs, planning for some social activities, such as a dinner. Too rigid a schedule interferes with participants achieving their secondary goals.

A schedule that is somewhat flexible and not too tightly arranged permits participants to learn from each other. In the coffee break example cited in Chapter 7, it can be noted that the nurse's remark that the best part of the conference was the coffee break suggests the value of interaction with colleagues.

SELECTION AND ORIENTATION OF FACULTY

Certain aspects of a short-term course may be taught by someone other than the regular faculty. When this is the case, teaching faculty are carefully selected and are usually chosen for their expert knowledge or skill in a specific content area.

Locating an appropriate person for a specific activity may be a challenge; since there is no *Who's Who in Nursing*, the program coordinator depends upon other sources of information. Suggestions for locating suitable part-time faculty are discussed in Chapter 13.

In whatever manner the faculty member is selected, it is desirable to have some recommendation of his ability to carry out the expected activity. Even with this precaution and with glowing reports of his abilities, occasional disappointments may occur, and the visiting faculty member fails to meet expectations.

To avoid needless disappointments the program coordinator assists the part-time faculty member in every possible way. A thorough explanation of the purposes and objectives of the conference is part of this orientation. The faculty member needs to have a detailed explanation of what is expected of him, the nature of the content, the type of presentation desired, and the amount of time allocated. To assist him in his preparation, it is helpful if he knows the number of expected enrollees and is given as much information about them as possible in advance of the program.

The part-time faculty member may make a more effective contribution if he attends the entire conference. If this is an expectation, it should be clearly understood when initial arrangements are made. A detailed copy of the program is sent to him, so he can see how his segment fits into the rest of the content and how it can best be coordinated with the presentations of others.

Although many preliminary arrangements are often made by telephone, a confirming letter is also required by visiting faculty. This letter verifies the arrangements for participation, and also includes details about the honorarium, the specific location of the conference, and information about hotel reservations. Travel suggestions may be appreciated, particularly if the conference is being held in an unusual location. Occasionally the plane ticket is secured and sent to the person. He may be asked to provide personal data (see Exhibit 9.3) and to notify the coordinator of any required teaching materials or audiovisual equipment.

Preliminary planning with the potential part-time faculty member includes a discussion of the financial arrangements for participation in the course. Institutions often have policies about the amount to be paid, but some flexibility is usually permitted. The honorarium may be large enough to cover the individual's fee and expenses; in other instances he may be paid a standard fee and be reimbursed for his actual expenses. Definite arrangements prevent later misunderstandings, and confirmation should be in writing.

Assistance to part-time faculty is always part of the coordinator's responsibilities. Additional support and reassurance may be required by the inexperienced person. Attention to detailed planning with the part-time faculty member assures a more effective presentation to the extent that it assists him in doing his best.

PUBLICITY

Selection of participants follows the completion of initial course planning. This requires that potential enrollees be informed about the course. Supportive service may be provided by the educational institution; in other settings, every detail must be managed by the faculty member responsible for the course.

Exhibit 9.3 SPEAKER INFORMATION SHEET

(A speaker information sheet can be used for promotional and publicity purposes and for introductions.)

Name: _____

Home address: _____

_____Phone:_____

Business address: _____

_____ Phone: _____

Position:_____

Past Experience:_____

_____

Education: _____

_____

_____

Publications:_____

_____

Date and time of presentation:_____

Place of meeting: _____

Title of presentation:_____

_____

(continued)

Exhibit 9.3 CONTINUED

Equipment and/or supplies needed: _____

Do you wish hotel reservations made for you?_____

Date and time of arrival: _____

Comments: _____

Even when public information service is available to the faculty member, he will need to develop content for descriptive fliers and brochures and provide information for news releases. Content includes all the pertinent information but should not be unnecessarily wordy. Accuracy is important.

Short-term courses may be publicized in many different ways: direct mailings of descriptive fliers or brochures; newspaper, radio, and television releases; news items in nursing publications; posters or other announcements in appropriate locations. In some instances only a direct mailing is used; at other times, all of these means may be used to publicize programs. Of all these approaches, direct mailing is usually the most effective one, so it is worthwhile to spend time and effort in designing an attractive and accurate brochure or flier to describe the offering.

A direct mailing is designed to go to individuals who are likely to attend. Cost is a factor in mailing since the brochure is sent to many more persons than can be expected to attend. If a suitable mailing list is not available, brochures are sent to institutions for posting on bulletin boards so that the information about the offering can be read by potential enrollees. Both a personal and an institutional mailing may be desirable.

Fliers and Brochures

The format used for describing any potential offering may vary from a simple mimeographed page to a very detailed printed brochure. Whatever the format used, it is carefully designed to provide accurate information in a way to encourage participation in the offering it describes.

Often preliminary announcements are mailed quite some time in advance of the date of the offering. This alerts interested persons to the scheduled dates and permits plans to be made for attending. A preliminary announcement usually suggests that those interested can request additional information (Exhibit 9.4). More detailed brochures are sent to those who indicate an interest in participating in the program.

News Releases

If assistance is not available, the faculty member or program coordinator may have to develop his own news releases. Even if an expert prepares the releases it is useful for faculty to be familiar with the preparation of news releases. They can then be more helpful to those who prepare them.

In any news release six questions are answered: who, what, where, when, why, and how. (See Fig. 9.5). The most useful releases are written in clear and simple language with short paragraphs. The important elements in the news releases are given first, with subsequent paragraphs progressively less important. If only a segment of the news release is used, then the less significant information at the end of the item is deleted.

Although educational institutions may have little difficulty in getting newspaper publicity, the release may not be used if it appears to be disguised advertising. Other reasons for failure to use releases are that they lack a local angle, are too long or too poorly written.

To assure use of a news item once it has been written, attention must be paid to a number of details. It is important to know the newspaper's deadlines and to plan accordingly. The date is placed at the top of the release. The source of information is given in the upper left hand corner, with a telephone number in case the editor wishes more information.

The appearance of a news release is also important. An original copy is sent to each newspaper. Copy is typed, double- or triple-spaced, on one side only of standard 8½ by 11 paper. The beginning of the story is started about one third of the way from the top of the page. Paragraphs are not continued from one page to another. Headlines are not included with the releases. If photographs are sent, attached to each is a complete caption, with full names and titles of those appearing in it, identified from left to right.

A sample news story for a refresher course is given on page 161. A news release for any type of short-term course would be similar.

Nursing Publications. News releases for the nursing publications may be developed for short term-courses with registration open to nurses from any

Exhibit 9.4   ADVANCE PRELIMINARY ANNOUNCEMENT

(An advance preliminary announcement helps potential enrollees plan for their participation in a forthcoming offering.)

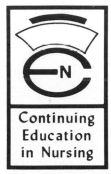

Continuing Education in Nursing

Preliminary Announcement
CRITICAL ISSUES IN CONTINUING EDUCATION IN NURSING
NATIONAL CONFERENCE ON CONTINUING EDUCATION IN NURSING
October 18-22, 1971
The University of Wisconsin Madison, Wisconsin

SPECIAL FEATURES:

● First day designed for those new to continuing education

● General sessions on philosophy of continuing education, implications for licensure, competencies of faculty, national and regional concerns

● Group discussions on critical issues in continuing education in nursing

● Optional "this-is-how-we-do-it" sessions

● Last day designed for discussion on organization and structure

For further information write to:

Department of Nursing
Health Sciences Unit
University Extension
The University of Wisconsin
610 Langdon Street
Madison, Wisconsin 53706

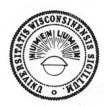

This conference is designed for registered nurses whose major responsibilities are in continuing education. The conference is planned to provide an opportunity for nurses involved in continuing nursing education to discuss issues and concerns, to share ideas and knowledge with others in comparable positions, and to learn about new developments in the field. It is designed for those nurses who are faculty members of a college or university, or on the in-service education staff of a medical center associated with an institution of higher learning, or on the staff of a Regional Medical Program.

National Conference on Continuing Education in Nursing. October 18-22, 1971.

Name _____

Address _____
                Street

_____
  City   State   Zip Code

Institution _____

Position _____

Figure 9.5   NEWS RELEASE INFORMATION FORM

(A news release information form outlines all the pertinent data about the course.)

To: Editor, Portage Daily News

From: Maribelle Smith, Public Information, University of Wisconsin-Extension, 262-0566

Who: Staff nurses in Wisconsin general hospitals

What: Are invited to attend a series of weekly seminars on planning patient care

Where: At the Wisconsin Center on campus of the University of Wisconsin-Madison

When: Tuesday evenings, 7-9 p.m. beginning April 6, 1972, for 8 sessions

Why: The sessions are one of a number of offerings provided by University Extension for upgrading patient care. This is the first of a series of 4 offerings planned over a two-year period.

How: The seminar is conducted by Gisella Jones, Asst. Prof. of Nursing, University of Wisconsin-Extension

Remarks: The seminar is sponsored by University Extension, the Wisconsin Nurses' Association, and the Wisconsin League for Nursing

---

location. National publications as well as state and district bulletins and newsletters are possibilities. A similar type of release may be used as for the newspapers although some nursing periodicals (*American Journal of Nursing, Journal of Continuing Education in Nursing*) have a regular format to follow. A copy of this format may be obtained from the publication.

Radio and Television.   Time for spot announcements on radio and television may be available as a public service, but such use of air time is often limited to that which appeals to a widespread audience. For this reason it may be difficult to get the time for announcements of nursing activities, but this possibility should not be overlooked.

Material for radio and television broadcasts must be very brief (see sample spot announcement on page 162. The station usually reserves the right to shorten and rewrite items to suit its time slots. Station managers prefer to get materials several days in advance of the broadcast during which the announcement will be made. For television, visual illustrations may be requested.

In addition to the use of spot announcements for publicizing programs, radio and television may be considered as a public relations tool for nursing. As an example of this use, some stations may be interested in knowing when certain well-known nursing leaders are appearing in a particular offering and may wish to arrange for an interview. If the content of an offering is newsworthy, small segments may be videotaped for a later news broadcast.

If the program coordinator does not have public information support, it may be useful for him to meet with the station manager personally. He will suggest approaches for cooperation with the station that will be mutually beneficial.

In addition to announcements about current offerings, other news items may be considered. Faculty can develop a sensitivity to newsworthy items and alert the staff of the appropriate news media. For example, community newspapers often use items about local nurses who participated in conferences. Picture feature stories are especially pertinent for clinical courses and refresher courses for inactive nurses. Human interest stories might be built around unusual experiences of nurses, which often come to light in short-term courses.

Conference Proceedings

Strictly speaking, conference proceedings cannot be classified as publicity, but the relationship is self-evident and so is discussed in this section. Editorial assistance and other administrative support may be available but the decision to publish proceedings is made by the conference staff, since considerable staff time is involved in preparation for publication.

Opinions differ over the value of conference proceedings so the decision about publishing them in any form must be carefully made. Distribution of proceedings may be limited to participants; in this case they are duplicated in the easiest possible way. Other proceedings may be widely promoted; then they are usually printed for distribution.

Ideally, decisions about distribution of proceedings are made before the conference is held. This advance decision is a difficult one, since the value of the content of a conference nor the results of a workshop cannot be anticipated in advance. In general, conference proceedings are more meaningful, and therefore most useful, to participants, so justification for wider distribution deserves careful consideration.

Planning for publication of proceedings includes ways of simplifying the process; for example, designating persons as recorders for selected segments of the conference or asking faculty members for prepared papers of their presentations. The entire conference may be tape recorded, but transcription is difficult, and advance arrangements are preferable. Securing the services of a stenotypist is another possibility but is expensive. Also, the presence of a stenotypist or a tape recorder may inhibit free discussion by participants.

Conference proceedings should always be edited. Verbatim proceedings include unnecessary social amenities ("Good morning. It's so wonderful to be with you in Milwaukee . . .") or even explanations about the location of meeting rooms. It is incredible that they are ever published this way, but it is not unusual to see such copy. Carefully edited proceedings distill the essence of the conference to make it meaningful to those unable to attend, but also to present an accurate, straightforward record for those who were there.

CONDUCT OF THE COURSE

Whatever the format for the short-term course, conference, workshop, institute, or clinical practicum, the ingredients for its successful execution are essentially the same. Clinical courses have an added component, and this will be discussed separately, but conducting the clinical course has many elements in common with other formats.

Selection of Enrollees

A basic principle of education identifies the value of starting where the learner is, and this suggests the need for some homogeneity in the knowledge base of participants. Unless this is recognized, much time is wasted by the more advanced student, while others are securing basic knowledge. In some learning experiences, such as the team conference, each person comes with some knowledge about the patient, and this common knowledge assists the learning process even though the learners have a variety of educational backgrounds. Sharing this knowledge, learning together, and working through solutions to nursing care problems promotes a cohesiveness that facilitates more effective team practice. The same thing is true of certain interprofessional learning experiences, provided the objectives are clearly identified and understood by all participants.

Conversely it may be impossible to provide a sound educational offering for a mix of practical nurses and registered nurses, or practicing and inactive nurses, or teachers who have little or no knowledge of educational theory and those who have a broad understanding. Prerequisites for enrolling in a course should be appropriate to its objectives, and when exceptions are made, the basis for the exception should be understood by the enrollee.

Selection of enrollees on the basis of the knowledge of the nurse is appropriate. In credit course offerings this is done by expecting the enrollee to meet certain prerequisites or to pass an examination showing that he possesses the required knowledge. In noncredit short-term courses, definite prerequisites or criteria are likewise often established as requirements for enrollment.

The establishment of enrollment criteria helps control extreme diversity within the group, and this facilitates teaching. Recognition of individual differences provides some flexibility, but great variation in the educational and experience backgrounds of enrollees may pose serious problems to the director of the course as he attempts to help learners meet their learning needs.

Criteria for enrollment in short-term courses often includes graduation from an accredited school of nursing, current registration to practice professional nursing, and a minimum amount of experience, as, for example, in a head nurse or supervisory position. In other courses more specific criteria must be met: current employment as an occupational health nurse, at least one year's experience in industry, a baccalaureate degree in nursing, and so on.

Presenting the Course

Various methods of teaching are discussed in Chapter 8, so this section will focus on general aspects rather than specific details of presentation. The success of a short-term course may depend as much on its general conduct as upon its content or the teaching methods used. Attitudes about the course may result from factors far removed from either.

Initial Impression. To a marked degree the success of a short term course depends upon the interaction of members of the group. With an awareness of the importance of such interaction, the course coordinator plans activities to promote group interface.

Early impressions may influence how enrollees react to a short-term course or to the sponsoring institution, and may include some items occurring before he appears at the conference center. Prompt attention to requests for information about the course will be noticed; so will the length of time taken to process his application form. Personal attention when he appears for the conference is also noted: the welcome he receives, the direction and assistance he is given in locating the proper room, introductions to other enrollees, and so on.

Helping group members get acquainted with each other may be done in many ways. Name tags are useful; so are table cards with each person's name written in letters sufficiently large to be seen across the room. For very large groups a combination of both the name tags and table cards helps enrollees learn each others' names, since name tags are worn at coffee breaks, lunch, and other places where table cards are not used.

Many times each person is asked to introduce himself at the beginning of the conference. A self-introduction may be somewhat uncomfortable for some persons, so it may be better for each person to introduce the person on his right or for enrollees to pair off and introduce each other. If either of these methods is used, time must be allotted for persons to get well enough acquainted to give the expected introduction. If each enrollee has a duplicated list of those present at the time introductions are made, he can learn their names more quickly.

Early attention to the creature comforts helps in the orientation to the conference and the setting. Unless they are very obvious, the locations of coat rooms, rest rooms, and reading rooms are given. Enrollees wish to know the time and location of coffee breaks and meals. If meals are to be taken away from the conference center, directions for finding dining facilities must be clear and explicit.

When conferees are on their own for certain meals, a list of names and addresses of restaurants is helpful. When the conference extends over a long period of time or is planned so there is considerable free time, a list of area recreational and educational facilities or entertainment possibilities is appreciated by enrollees.

A Climate for Learning. The concern for enrollees as expressed early in the course helps establish a climate conducive to learning. A warm, accepting, helpful attitude initiated by faculty at the beginning and extending throughout the entire course, contributes to the learning process. Each enrollee's feeling of acceptance by faculty members helps assure the learners' acceptance of each other and thus contributes to their learning from each other.

Faculty expectations also contribute to the learning process. If enrollees clearly understand what is expected of them, they will put forth an early effort to comply, particularly if the assignment is accompanied by an adequate explanation of the value of the activity to the students' learning. Teachers may underestimate the student's willingness to put forth the effort to learn and so unwittingly contribute to his failure.

Many practicing nurses belittle their own abilities. In part this may be the result of a combination of factors: an education that stifled creativity and fostered dependency, and employment in settings that discouraged individual initiative and provided little recognition. In their early continuing education experiences, many nurses may require an unusual amount of support and reassurance.

Group Work. With the exception of the institute, short-term courses are built around group participation. They are based on the concept that each participant has knowledge and experience that contributes to the learning of other members of the group.

Participants in short-term courses usually have had a variety of group experiences, although not necessarily successful ones. These experiences include nursing team conferences, faculty or staff meetings, committee work, and various types of community group involvement.

Faculty members, too, have had a variety of group experiences. Effective group leadership requires some knowledge of and practice in using informal group techniques. Courses in communication skills, leadership techniques, and group discussion are sponsored by many different institutions and organizations, and inexperienced faculty members can be encouraged to enroll. Much has been written on the subject of group work; a number of these references are listed at the end of the chapter.

Clinical Courses

The graduate of today's school of nursing may lack some of the clinical expertise of his counterpart of some years ago but may know much more, as a result of the rapid expansion of knowledge which demanded changes in nursing curriculum. Among these changes has been an increase in the scientific bases, but a decrease in the amount of clinical practice for the student. Thus the new graduate has a depth of knowledge but is not a polished practitioner.

Many nurses feel a need to add depth to both their clinical knowledge and their nursing skill. Carefully designed clinical courses can help meet this need. Planning a series or sequence of courses contributes to a depth of knowledge.

Courses in rehabilitation nursing may be cited as examples of these clinical courses. As knowledge of rehabilitation expanded, it became apparent that the principles could be applied to the care of many patients if nurses understood these principles. Short-term courses in rehabilitation nursing were established at Boston University in 1962; similar action by a number of educational institutions followed. The graduate program in rehabilitation nursing has been offered at Boston University since 1955, and to some extent the sequence of events is the reverse of the usual pattern. Often short-term, noncredit courses are established, and having proved their worth, gain academic respectability. Although the principles of rehabilitation nursing are now offered as graduate courses in nursing in many institutions, short-term courses on this content continue to meet a need.

The value of the clinical course was further dramatized with the advent of the coronary care unit. To provide adequate care to patients, practicing nurses needed a depth of knowledge not presented in their basic educational programs. Once established, coronary care units mushroomed all across the country, but nurses employed in them were not prepared for the responsibilities expected of them.

To help meet these learning needs, in 1967 the Division of Nursing of the U.S. Public Health Service promoted the development of short term courses on coronary care. These courses, from four to six weeks in length, were established in twelve different institutions, in strategic locations throughout the country. Courses were supported by federal funds, which included stipends for those who attended.

Fewer coronary care courses now receive federal support, but the need for such instruction persists, and courses designed on the pattern of the original models continue to be offered by some institutions. Occasionally the content has been broadened to include both coronary and intensive care.

In general, clinical courses are designed in areas of nursing where in-depth preparation is not possible in the basic curriculum, or where the expansion of knowledge has altered nursing practice extensively. Courses may be provided to help nurses gain skill in the care of neurological patients, emotionally disturbed children, and patients with renal disease, to name a few additional examples.

Content for the clinical course must be carefully planned. It is designed to add to the nurse's depth of knowledge, and planned experiences permit the application of this knowledge to nursing practice.

The selection of the practice field is of utmost importance for an effective clinical course. This includes an adequate number of patients, a supportive nursing and medical staff, a climate conducive to learning, and a satisfactory physical facility, including ready access to conference and other meeting rooms.

Learning experiences are designed to build on the nurse's previous knowledge. Since enrollees come with a variety of educational and experiential backgrounds, it takes time and considerable skill to plan a course meaningful to all enrollees. The practicum provides an opportunity for individualized learning experiences, and the sequence of these experiences is carefully worked out.

The provision of a wide variety of learning tools can assist in meeting individual learner's needs. Access to a wide variety of self-study materials, study carrels, books, and periodicals contributes to this aspect of learning. Exposure of the learner to the literature of his area of nursing practice is of special importance, since one of the objectives of any clinical course is to encourage the nurse to continue self-directed study after the course is completed.

Evaluation

Evaluation is recognized as an integral part of every short-term course. Determining the means of evaluation is part of course planning. The principles of evaluation are discussed in detail in Chapter 14.

REFERENCES

Adult Education Association of the U.S.A.: "How to Lead Discussions," Leadership Pamphlet No. 1, The Association, Chicago, 1955.

_____: "Planning Better Programs," Leadership Pamphlet No. 2, The Association, Chicago, 1955.

_____: "Understanding How Groups Work," Leadership Pamphlet No. 4, The Association, Chicago, 1955.

_____: "How to Teach Adults," Leadership Pamphlet No. 5, The Association, Chicago, 1955.

_____: "Conducting Workshops and Institutes," Leadership Pamphlet No. 9, The Association, Chicago, 1955.

_____: "Conferences That Work," Leadership Pamphlet No. 11, The Association, Chicago, 1955.

Beckhard, Richard: *Conference Planning*, National Training Laboratories, National Education Association, Washington, D.C., 1962.

Bergevin, Paul, Dwight Morris, and Robert M. Smith: *Adult Education Procedures*, The Seabury Press, New York, 1963.

Elfenbein, Julien: *Editor's Manual*, The American Journal of Nursing Company, New York, 1970, Chap. 5-8.

Gessner, Quentin H.: Planning Educational Conferences, *Adult Lead.*, 18(2): 45-46; 65-66, 1969.

Kindler, Herbert S.: *Organizing the Technical Conference*, Rheinhold Publishing Company, New York, 1970.

Knowles, Malcolm: "Program Planning for Adults and Learners," *Adult Lead.*, 15(8): 267-268; 278-279, 1967.

Knowles, Malcolm, and Hulda Knowles: *Introduction to Group Dynamics*, Association Press, New York, 1959.

Lindeman, Carol: "University in a Suitcase," *Amer. J. Nurs.*, 66(4): 781-782, 1966.

Nusinoff, Janet Ryen: "A Structural Approach to Inservice Education," *J. Contin. Educ. Nurs.*, 1(4): 21-27, 1970.

"Publicity Handbook: A Guide for Publicity Chairmen," *Consumer Relations*, The Sperry and Hutchinson Company, 3003 East Kemper Road, Cincinnati, Ohio, 45241, 1965.

Rindt, Kenneth E.: *Handbook for Coordinators of Management and Other Adult Education Programs*, University Extension, University of Wisconsin, Commerce Department, Management Institute, Madison, Wis., 1968.

Schweer, Jean E.: "Continuing Education Climatology," *J. Nurs. Admin.*, 1(1): 45-48, 1971.

White, John M., "Checklist for a Workshop or Conference," Oklahoma Regional Medical Program, 828 Northeast Fifteenth Street, Oklahoma City, Oklahoma, 73104, n.d.

Zelko, Harold P.: *Successful Conference and Discussion Techniques*, McGraw-Hill Book Company, New York, 1957.

10

Refresher courses for inactive nurses

Refresher courses for inactive nurses were among the earliest types of continuing education in nursing; the history of this development is discussed in Chapter 2. This chapter is designed to provide guidelines for instructors responsible for planning and conducting these courses.

The need for refresher courses to keep pace with nursing service demands is likely to continue for some time. Eventually this need may change as increasing numbers of married women continue employment, and as more opportunities for part-time work become available.

Every nurse who has been inactive for any length of time knows that returning to employment requires considerable adjustment. During periods of inactivity, nurses often make no effort to keep in touch with their profession or are unable to locate resources for keeping updated, so filling in gaps in knowledge and practice is required.

To some extent the old myth, "Once a nurse, always a nurse" has perpetuated the idea that returning to practice is relatively simple. Schools of nursing are beginning to instill in students the concept of lifelong learning; inactive nurses are beginning to appreciate the need for planning and preparation for an eventual return to practice. More imaginative approaches in helping these nurses keep professionally informed would also facilitate their return to nursing.

Increased opportunities for part-time employment would encourage many nurses to keep in touch professionally and would hasten their return to the full-time work force. Better utilization of the part-time nurse would result in increased job satisfaction, which in itself encourages longer periods of employment.

At best a refresher course is only the beginning step toward a return to practice. No course ever replaces an adequate orientation to a specific position in nursing or supportive supervision throughout the early employment period. The nurse who returns to practice needs and wants assistance as she begins her first position. Unless she is assured of such assistance, she may decide against returning to practice.

Several studies of nurses who have been employed following completion of refresher courses indicate that many work only for short periods of time. This may relate to the quality or effectiveness of the course, but it also suggests inadequate supervision and orientation to the first position, and perhaps lack of sufficient care in job placement. Frequently the returning nurse is placed in a position of considerable responsibility before she is ready for it.

Assistance is always required by the nurse who returns to employment. The interest shown by other employees also contributes to the likelihood of her remaining in the position.

WHO IS THE INACTIVE NURSE?

Many challenges await the instructor who teaches inactive nurses, for usually this group is a heterogeneous one. Although prospective candidates are screened to provide for some homogeneity, differences in education and work experience are always present. These differences will force the instructor to use a wide variety of teaching methods and to individualize instruction wherever appropriate.

One cannot make generalizations about inactive nurses, for many individual differences are found in any particular group. In teaching them and in working with inactive nurses, these individual differences must be sought and teaching planned around them. It is helpful, though, to be aware of certain recurrent characteristics.

Almost without exception the inactive nurse has heavy home and family responsibilities and this is usually her main reason for not working. When she attends the refresher course she brings her home concerns with her: Is the baby-sitter a responsible one? What to have for dinner tonight? How to arrange for the plumber to come?

The inability to solve home problems may keep the nurse from attending the course. Interestingly, many nurses have found that while participating in a refresher course they have learned how to plan better and how to get more family involvement in household tasks. If she finds the home situation manageable the nurse is then encouraged to seek employment upon the completion of the course.

Inactive nurses enrolled in refresher courses come from a variety of educational programs: baccalaureate, hospital diploma, and two-year associate degree programs. In any group there may be individuals who have graduated from similar types of programs, but if there is a great gap in the years when they were graduated, there will be major differences in the content and methods of teaching used. Many of these nurses have had some additional education beyond their basic training program.

These nurses also have had a variety of experiences, both in length and type. The majority, but not all, have had staff experience following graduation. Although there are some exceptions, in general the nurse who has had substantial experience before she left the practice of her profession will find it easier to make the transition back to employment.

The teacher of the refresher course will find it helpful to have as much information about each enrollee as possible since this assists her in planning the course. This information is usually secured by means of an application blank and a personal interview.

Susan Adams: A Returning Nurse

Although inactive nurses share some common characteristics it is difficult to identify a typical inactive nurse. Rather one must look at the individual nurse and assess her peculiar learning needs.

Susan Adams, 35, has not practiced her profession for twelve years. She left nursing when she was pregnant with her first child. Now the mother of three youngsters, Sally, 12, George, 10, and Patty, 7, Mrs. Adams leads a busy and varied life. She teaches Sunday School, is a den mother, vice-president of the PTA, active in the League of Women Voters, and belongs to a bridge club and a bowling league.

Even with all her activities Susan felt the urge to return to nursing ever since Patty entered kindergarten. But the critical articles about hospitals and nursing care in the women's magazines and some of the stories she hears over the bridge table discouraged her.

Six months ago she learned that a refresher course was to be offered in a local hospital so she promptly enrolled. While taking the course she discovered that she could organize her personal life more efficiently; she even found that Sally seemed better-natured now that she had more home responsibilities.

Susan found the new developments in nursing exciting and challenging, but she was also reassured to learn that many of the basic principles of nursing care still applied. She discovered that she was now more able to be supportive to patients; she had lived through some difficult times herself, and found that her personal experiences gave her a new and deeper understanding of others' problems.

Susan was pleased with the new nursing books; she was quite surprised to learn that several of these books could be found in the public library. She subscribed to a nursing periodical, and several of the members of her refresher class decided to meet once a month as a journal club to discuss articles in current periodicals.

After she completed the course Susan decided to seek employment. Neither of the local hospitals were employing part-time nurses at the time she applied, but she was sure that full-time employment was more than she could manage. She next applied at a private nursing home, and found that they would be happy to have her two days a week. Although somewhat difficult, the work has been very satisfying to her, and she has found that occasionally she can work an additional day when needed.

In evaluating her experience, Susan thinks that the transition from housewife to nurse would have been even more difficult had she waited longer. She has had to make some adjustments; she has given up bridge club, but she is often able to substitute for an absent member. Her household is a little more hectic, perhaps, as she hurries off to the 7 o'clock tour of duty, but she feels her return to practice has resulted in some deep personal satisfaction to herself, and she is pleased that her family feels she is making an important contribution to the community.

Not all returning nurses find satisfying positions, and the challenges in the modern hospital setting may be so overwhelming that some cannot cope with the situation. However, if the refresher course is well-planned and well-taught many inactive nurses renew their initial enthusiasm and remain in practice for long periods of time.

PLANNING FOR REFRESHER COURSES

State-wide or regional planning for refresher courses appears to be most logical, but frequently decisions about offering these courses are made at a local level. However the decision is made, it should follow careful study to determine the need for the course, whether there will be sufficient enrollment to justify the cost and effort, and whether there are suitable positions available to the nurses who complete the course.

Local planning committees vary in composition but may include representatives from the hospitals and other health agencies in the community, district nurses' associations, hospital and medical associations, schools of nursing, departments of health and education, employment security office and the health planning council, directors of nursing and administrators of hospitals and nursing homes, and inactive nurses. Such a planning committee can assist in determining the need for the course in the community and if employment opportunities exist. The committee can also assist in broad planning for course content, suggesting suitable instructors, assistance with promotion, and evaluation of the course.

It may not always be possible, but publicizing plans for several years in advance is helpful to the individual nurse. It is easier for her to make a decision if she knows when and where courses will be offered in the future.

Location of the Course

In the planning of any refresher course, careful consideration is given to its location. If there is only one hospital in the community this is not a difficult decision. If there is more than one, careful planning may be required to decide upon any particular institution or to plan ways of utilizing all available resources. In selecting facilities, clinical resources must be carefully evaluated for their adequacy for teaching purposes. Administrative support and interest by the nursing staff are also important considerations.

An accessible library is another requirement. The assistance of a librarian in collecting appropriate materials contributes substantially to the success of the course. Enrollees should be encouraged to use all the resources of the library, including self-study materials, and be permitted to borrow books for home study.

If the course is offered in an institution without a library, additional efforts are required to locate necessary reference materials and appropriate space to store and display them. Easy access to materials will promote further study by participants, but relearning the use of the library is an integral part of the course.

A unit library is also useful; this enables the enrollees to locate pertinent information while caring for patients. Unit libraries include a medical dictionary, a text on drugs (or *Physician's Desk Reference*), procedure and policy manuals, and current nursing texts.

Funding the Course

The decisions about funding the course should be made early in the planning period. Some refresher courses have been supported by federal funds, such as those provided by the 1965 amendments to the Manpower Development and Training Act and through regional medical programs. Others have been funded through private sources. Many are financed, at least in part, by charging a tuition fee.

A tuition fee rarely deters the nurse who wishes to enroll. It may serve to encourage her to take a course since fee payment may relieve her of an obligation to work at its completion. There are other values in having the nurse pay an individual fee: since she has a personal investment in the course, she may take it more seriously and put forth greater efforts to learn.

Hospitals frequently offer refresher courses as a community service. Under these circumstances a fee may or may not be charged. If there is a fee it may be refunded if the nurse returns to practice in the hospital offering the course.

Costs of programs vary, but in determining tuition fees, consideration should be given to the salary for the instructor, textbooks, film rental and other teaching supplies, telephone and mailing expenses for promotional materials.

Costs to the individual enrollee must also be considered. These involve expenses for uniforms, shoes, hose; costs for relicensure; transportation and parking; and, for many enrollees, child care and housekeeping services.

Publicity

Advance notice that the refresher course will be offered gives the nurse time to arrange her home affairs, purchase uniforms, and take care of other necessary details, such as securing current state licensure. Arrangements for child care and transportation may also take time.

Locating Inactive Nurses.   Information which determines the need for the course is best obtained from inactive nurses themselves, but locating these nurses may be difficult. Newspaper releases and radio and television spot announcements help acquaint inactive nurses of the possibility of the course being offered. These announcements may be made several months before the course will be taught.

Directors of nursing in hospitals or nursing homes frequently have lists of names of inactive nurses. The state board of nursing is another possible source, although its list may not be completely up to date.

If there is a school of nursing in the community, its alumni association may have a list of inactive nurses or may be willing to publish an appropriate item in its newsletter. The district nurses' association may have a list of inactive nurses. Announcements at nursing meetings are also appropriate since practicing nurses often have friends who are inactive.

Posters in supermarkets, laundromats, libraries, and banks may be useful in the search for inactive nurses. Notices in church bulletins might also be considered.

Publicizing the Course.   After the decision has been made to offer the course the detailed information about it is distributed, preferably six weeks in advance. Essentially, the same routes can be used again: newspaper, radio, television; nursing association announcements and newsletters; posters in hospitals, nursing homes, and buildings where nurses are likely to be found.

Preparing news releases is discussed in detail in Chapter 9; a sample release for a refresher course is shown in Exhibit 10.1. The news release covers all the information the inactive nurse needs to know to make a decision about enrolling. This information, in journalistic terms, includes the who, what, when, where, why, and how of the course, detailed in Exhibit 10.2.

The best promotional device is mailing a descriptive flier to the prospective enrollee. These names and addresses are secured from the early publicity. Fliers include all the information in the news release plus other significant details, such as the amount of clinical practice, suggestions about securing licensure, recom-

Exhibit 10.1   SAMPLE NEWS RELEASE FOR
REFRESHER COURSE IN NURSING

(The news release for a refresher course gives the potential
enrollees the necessary information about the offering.)

Department of Nursing
Centerville College
Mrs. Henrietta Martin   FOR IMMEDIATE RELEASE
Monroe, Wisconsin
Phone: 262-0566

Inactive professional nurses in Monroe and the surrounding area
will be able to update their knowledge and prepare for a return to
practice with a six-week refresher course to begin March 6. The course
is sponsored by Centerville College and Monroe Memorial Hospital.
The noncredit course will be offered Mondays through Fridays,
from 8:30 A.M. to 3:00 P.M. Classes and clinical practice will be held at
the hospital.
The course will be taught by Mrs. Marie Nelson, R.N., assistant
professor of nursing, Centerville College, assisted by Marion Miller,
R.N., and Mrs. Elizabeth Adams, R.N., both nursing supervisors at
Memorial Hospital.
Enrollment will be limited to 20, and preference will be given to
those nurses planning to return to practice. Current registration or a
permit to practice nursing in Wisconsin is required for participation.
For further information and application blanks, write Mrs.
Henrietta Martin, Department of Nursing, Centerville College, Monroe,
or call 262-0566.

mended textbooks, uniform requirements, parking. Enrollees usually want additional information about instructional staff, such as their education and past experience. Any prerequisites, such as a physical examination, are stated in the flier.

When a telephone number is given for further information, the person answering should not only have all the essential information but should also be as helpful and supportive as possible to the caller. The insecure nurse may have a difficult time deciding to take the course, so she needs all available information to help her make the decision.

Exhibit 10.2   RADIO SPOT ANNOUNCEMENT

(Brief news releases, such as radio spot announcements, alert potential enrollees to future course offerings. Advance information assists them in planning for their participation in the course.)

Time: 20 seconds

Inactive nurses in the Monroe area will be offered a nursing refresher course by Centerville College beginning next fall. It is important, however, that possible enrollees make their interest known at this time.

The course is designed to acquaint inactive nurses with current trends in nursing and newer methods and techniques of nursing practice.

Interested inactive nurses should contact Mrs. Marie Nelson, Centerville College, Monroe, 262-0566.

Selecting Enrollees

Inactive nurses may enroll in a refresher course for a variety of reasons, so many factors may enter into determining admission to the course. The final decision is usually made by the instructor, but it is helpful if more than one person is involved, particularly if there are any troublesome aspects regarding enrollment.

Much information about enrollees can be secured through a completed application blank. This form includes personal information: name, address, telephone number, age, marital status, number and ages of children. It also includes information about enrollee's education and work experience: school of nursing, additional education, employment history, length of inactivity. Plans for future employment may be included. Information about licensure status is requested.

The age and health of the nurse may cause potential concern. A health statement from the individual's physician about her physical condition is usually required and may be helpful in determining admission to the course. Age limitations may be placed on enrollment, relating to the likelihood of the nurse's return to practice as well as her ability to practice, but individual factors ought to be carefully considered.

Current state registration—or a permit to practice, if the applicant is in the process of securing licensure—is required for participation in the course. If the applicant is not currently registered, she is directed to the state board of nursing for information about registration procedure.

The individual interview is important in deciding upon acceptance. The interview should obviously be held where privacy is assured. It permits securing more detailed information about the person's education and experience than is available on the application blank. Attitudes about nursing and work can be identified. The candidate's questions about the course can be answered in more detail. Reasons for taking the course and the applicant's intent to practice are also discussed.

In some situations it may be appropriate to limit enrollment to only those nurses who plan to return to practice, but even when a hospital is providing the course at no cost to the individual, there may be reasons to admit some nurses who do not plan immediate employment. The provision of a refresher course is a community service and, thus, providing the course may be seen as an educational responsibility of the hospital. The nurse may be better able to perform her citizenship obligations as a result of taking the course. For example, she will be much better informed about current nursing education and can more effectively interpret modern nursing to prospective candidates for schools of nursing.

Criteria for enrollment are best established in the planning stage for the course. Enrollees should be familiar with these criteria.

Instructional Staff

Planning also involves the selection of appropriate faculty to teach the course. Instructors for refresher courses are carefully selected for their teaching abilities and their knowledge of current nursing practice. They must have an understanding of the older learner and appreciate that this nurse has special contributions to make to her profession.

Requirements for the teaching staff will vary in different locations and will depend upon the policies of the institution offering the course. A baccalaureate degree and some teaching experience are minimal qualifications.

Instructors in these programs must have a good understanding of the needs of nurses who have been inactive, as well as a knowledge of the principles of adult education. The teacher must understand that many inactive nurses, although vaguely aware of such things as the new mathematics, may not be familiar with modern teaching approaches and will need encouragement to participate in class discussion or in using the new educational media.

The understanding teacher will be sympathetic to the adjustment the inactive nurse must make to present-day nursing practice. It may be helpful, though certainly not required, if the teacher herself has been inactive for some time.

Flexibility in planning and teaching is requisite, as is the teacher's ability to assist these students to regain their self-confidence. The instructor must be able to help each nurse discover her particular strengths, regain old skills, and develop new ones. He encourages questions and is available to respond to them or to find resources to seek answers, as well as to provide necessary reassurance.

Past teaching experience is useful, although the instructor who has previously taught only in undergraduate programs will need to modify his teaching so that it is acceptable to registered nurses. The teacher needs the ability to help these nurses relate their previous experience to present day practice and also to build on this experience in teaching the course. Skill is required to help these students give up formerly held ideas which apply no longer and to redevelop an interest in and excitement for learning.

A familiarity with nursing as it is practiced today is necessary, as is a deep understanding of current developments in the whole field of health. To help students appreciate the significance of these developments, a knowledge of the social and economic trends influencing the health professions is essential.

Another prerequisite for the instructor is that he have an awareness of the many learning resources available to the nurse today. Helping enrollees locate these resources and learn how to use them is an integral part of the course. The effective teacher also motivates students to continue their learning after the course is completed.

For the returning nurse the concept of continuing education for professional practice may be a new idea. The instructor can be of no greater service than to encourage these nurses to continue their learning efforts after the course ends. These students are eager to learn—the teacher has only to capture the zest and enthusiasm they bring with them to the course.

COURSE CONTENT

The refresher course is designed to update the inactive nurse with regard to current developments in nursing. Although courses are frequently offered in hospitals, the teacher must emphasize that nursing is practiced in many settings today. Identifying the role of the nurses outside of the hospital is an important aspect of any refresher course.

Course content is based upon the health needs in the particular community, as well as upon a consideration of the major health problems in the country. Helping the enrollee understand significant trends in nursing is an integral part of the course.

Since the refresher course is based on a knowledge of community expectations, each course is individually designed. It may be helpful to study outlines of courses offered elsewhere but an effective course has its own unique design.

Obviously content must be carefully selected within the time limitations of the particular course. Refresher courses vary in length, although most of them range from 80 to 160 hours. Approximately half of this time is devoted to clinical practice. In addition to formal classes and demonstrations, time is allocated for patient-care conferences, usually immediately following the student's clinical experience each day.

Determining Objectives

As with any type of educational offering, content is selected on the basis of the objectives for the course, so course planning begins with a determination of objectives. Course objectives are discussed in Chapter 6, and the reader will find it useful to refer to that material.

Many teachers find writing objectives difficult but, to reduce the process to its simplest terms, the objectives answer the question "What are we trying to do?" Obviously, then, the major objective of any refresher course is to facilitate the return of the inactive nurse to practice. Identifying more specific objectives helps to determine course content. For example, if an objective relates to regaining skill in the pre- and post-operative care of selected surgical patients, this content will be included in the course, and some clinical experience will be provided to assure that enrollees have the opportunity to regain the skill stated in the objective. Carefully selected objectives assist in the evaluation process, so care in the determination of course objectives is time well spent.

Selecting Learning Experiences

The determination of content for classes is no easy matter, for the time is limited and the instructor is tempted to teach as much as he possibly can. Usually it is best to design the course with a specific focus such as medical and surgical nursing, recognizing that the nurse who plans to return to another area of clinical practice will need additional assistance.

Content is planned in as logical a sequence as possible, building on the knowledge of the enrollee. Careful planning can help avoid wasting the students' time in reteaching those aspects of care that are remembered. Nurses remember how to make beds and give baths and administer enemas though they will need updating on new adaptations, such as disposable equipment. Additional references, self-teaching devices, and other related tools may be suggested for those enrollees for whom a basic review of certain areas may be indicated.

In determining content there may be a temptation to select those aspects of nursing which are totally new, unique, and unfamiliar, and this is the kind of content enrollees frequently request. It is not appropriate to spend a lot of the limited course time on kidney dialysis, coronary care, or organ transplants, when the nurse will not be returning to the care of these patients immediately if at all. Usually it is sufficient to give a brief description with an explanation that such specialized nursing care requires more preparation than can be obtained in a

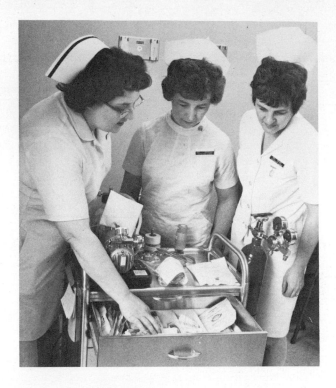

Figure 10-1   Clinical practice is an essential part of any
refresher course. Here enrollees are intro-
duced to the emergency cart. (*University
of Wisconsin-Extension*)

refresher course. Available readings on subjects of special interest are also useful
for the nurse who wishes more information.

When refresher courses are offered by a hospital there is a temptation to
teach nursing procedures as practiced in that setting, rather than to emphasize
underlying principles. Refresher courses are offered as a community service, and
as such, their content should not be limited to that appropriate for only one
employment setting.

Clinical Experience

Practice for the enrollee on the hospital unit is an integral part of the
course (Fig. 10-1). Experiences appropriate to meeting the objectives of the
course are selected.

Adequate supervision is necessary for a successful course and the person assigned this responsibility should have no other duties during the time enrollees are having their clinical practice. Time for planning appropriate clinical experiences is also necessary. In most courses the person teaching the major portion of the course will also be responsible for supervising the clinical practice of some of the enrollees. This depends on the length of the course each week, for he must be permitted adequate time for class preparation.

The number of enrollees assigned to each clinical instructor will vary. In planning, the student's abilities, the physical plant, and the degree of illness of the patient must be considered.

The hospital unit selected for this practice should have patients who present a variety of nursing problems. It is helpful if the nursing staff is a stable one; adequate staffing of the unit helps assure that enrollees will see examples of good nursing care.

The interest of the nursing staff, professional and auxiliary, can contribute to the success of any refresher course. A nursing staff that is helpful and supportive to the inactive nurses will not only help to make the course a success but also encourage the nurse to return to practice.

Interest of the nursing staff does not come about by accident but is the result of careful planning. The entire staff should be informed of plans before the course is offered. The attitude of the head nurse towards the enrollees can be a decisive factor in the treatment afforded them.

In determining appropriate clinical assignments, the background of the students, their needs and interests, and their previous experience are considered. Individual planning is required, for not all inactive nurses can handle the same assignments. Conferring with the student about her needs and interests helps provide a meaningful experience.

Enriching Experiences

Learning experiences available in the community can enhance the course. Since time is limited these experiences must be carefully evaluated for their appropriateness to the curriculum offered. Resources will vary from one community to the other.

Examples of these enriching experiences include a carefully planned tour of a nursing home or extended care facility; this may be new to the inactive nurse. A visit to a rehabilitation center can help identify a new concept of care, as can a trip to an institution for the retarded or to a mental health center. Dramatic changes have occurred in the care of the mentally ill, so a field trip to a psychiatric hospital may be valuable if the institution offering the course does not have a psychiatric unit.

Meeting a public health nurse in the classroom or at the agency can help identify her role in the provision of health services. The concept of continuity of care may be a new one to many enrollees, so this can be amplified by the community health nurse.

Teaching Aids

Textbooks designed for inactive nurses are now available and are useful teaching adjuncts. Current nursing and medical books, periodicals, reprints, pamphlets and monographs contribute much to learning if carefully selected.

A reading list or syllabus assists the enrollee in the learning process. Sometimes nurses ask for this information in advance of the course, to permit initial preparation. Inactive nurses have a wide range of interests, so extensive reading lists can help meet these individual needs.

Many additional aids are now available for use in the teaching of nursing. These include films, filmstrips, slides, audiotapes, transparencies, programmed units, charts, models, and photographs. These must be reviewed and carefully selected for their appropriateness in meeting the course objectives.

In addition, the imaginative instructor can develop his own teaching materials, such as transparencies for overhead projectors, flip charts, posters, and photographs or slides. Cleverly designed bulletin boards are useful to illustrate class content, and to stimulate interest in a particular subject.

Suggested bibliographic and resource materials are listed in many of the references given at the end of this chapter. Suggested course content is included in several of these references.

Final Steps

After the objectives are selected, course content determined, appropriate references, aids and resources selected, the course outline is developed. A class schedule is next designed, and a copy of this schedule is given to each enrollee. This helps set the stage for learning, since the enrollee knows what to expect in advance of each learning experience. A suggested outline for the first week is given in Exhibit 10.3.

EVALUATION

Evaluation is an integral part of the refresher course, and plans for evaluation should be included in the general planning for the course. Evaluation in any refresher course includes two aspects: the evaluation of the learner's performance and the determination of the effectiveness of the course. Observation of the learner's performance in clinical practice helps determine the effectiveness of the course; it may also serve as a guide to later employment.

Information from employers of inactive nurses can help evaluate the effectiveness of the refresher course preparation of the nurse after a return to employment. These are most useful if the information can be secured from the nurse's supervisor.

Exhibit 10.3   REFRESHER COURSE IN NURSING—SAMPLE SCHEDULE FOR FIRST WEEK

(Content scheduled may vary from one course to another depending on the needs of the group.)

Time	Monday	Tuesday
8:30 A.M.	Introductions Introduction to the course Enrollee expectations Facilities: parking, cafeteria, lounge, lockers, library Pretest and discussion Trends in nursing	Introduction to unit personnel Ward walk: meeting and observing patients; physical layout; location of supplies and equipment; procedure and policy manuals; unit library Assignments to patient care; study nursing care plans
11:30 A.M.	Changing patterns of health care	Patient care conference and discussion of observations on the unit
12:30 P.M.	Lunch	Lunch
1:30 P.M.	Brief tour of the hospital and discussion	Nursing service today; role of various workers; the health team Changing patterns of nursing education
3:00- 3:30 P.M.	Discuss next day's assignment	Discuss next day's assignment

(continued)

Exhibit 10.3 CONTINUED

Wednesday	Thursday

Patient care:
  Study nursing care plans
  Vital signs; use of
    electronic equipment
  Note medications and
    review them
  Review physician's order
    sheet
  Note safety measures
	Patient care:
	  Study nursing care plans
	  Note medications and
	    review them
	  Positioning and range of
	    motion exercises
	  Assisting in and out of
	    bed

Patient care conference
  and discussion of
  clinical assignment
	Patient care conference
	  and discussion of
	  clinical assignment

Lunch	Lunch

Body mechanics and posi-
  tioning of the patient
Range of motion exercises
  (Film, demonstration and
  return demonstration)
	Tour of central supply
	  department:
	    Disposables
	    Prepackaged items
	    New equipment

Discuss next day's
  assignment
	Summary and review of
	  first week's activities

The principles of evaluation of continuing education programs discussed in Chapter 14 apply to refresher courses. As previously discussed, clearly stated objectives assist in evaluation. In almost all instances one of the objectives will relate to return to practice. This can be simply measured by a telephone survey or brief questionnaire. If more extensive information is desired, a more elaborate questionnaire may be used (see Exhibit 10.4). The survey can be done at any time following completion of the course. Subsequent surveys may also be desirable to determine how long the enrollee continued employment.

Exhibit 10.4

REFRESHER COURSE QUESTIONNAIRE

Refresher Course _____

Enrollee # _____

Name _____

Address _____

Marital Status: Single _____ Married _____ Widowed _____ Divorced or Separated _____ Year of Birth _____

Number of Children _____ Age of Youngest Child _____

1. At the time you took The University of Wisconsin refresher course in nursing you were: (Please Check One)
   Inactive _____ Employed part time _____ Employed full time _____ Employed at something other than nursing _____

   If employed, what type of work? _____

2. If you were not employed at nursing at the time you took the refresher course, how many years had you been inactive? _____ years.

3. Are you now employed in nursing? (Check One)
   No, not working now _____ Yes, full time _____ Yes, part time _____ If part time, number of hours per week _____

4. Answer these questions IF YOU ARE NOT NOW EMPLOYED IN NURSING.
   Were you employed at any time following completion of the refresher course? Yes _____ No _____
   If "yes" for how long? _____
   Check the one main reason that you are not now working (circle any others that are also appropriate):
   _____ a. Employment opportunities not available locally.
   _____ b. Employers cannot use the working hours I am available.
   _____ c. I cannot make suitable arrangements for the care of my child (or children).
   _____ d. Transportation not available.
   _____ e. The salary I would get would not make it worthwhile.
   _____ f. I am unable to secure necessary domestic help.
   _____ g. My health does not permit my return to active practice.
   _____ h. I prefer to be a homemaker.
   _____ i. My husband does not want me to work.
   _____ j. I believe that a mother should be in the home while children are young.
   _____ k. I am not interested in nursing.
   _____ l. Other (Specify) _____
   Are you employed for pay at something other than nursing? Yes _____ No _____

   If "yes" please indicate type of employment _____
   Do you anticipate employment in nursing sometime in the future? Yes _____ No _____ Maybe _____

5. Answer these questions only if you were INACTIVE at the time you took the course and are NOW OR HAVE BEEN EMPLOYED ANYTIME SINCE TAKING THE COURSE.
   Did you receive an adequate orientation to the hospital (or agency) when beginning employment?
   Yes _____ No _____

   If "no" please explain: _____
   _____
   _____

   Did you find that you were better prepared to perform nursing duties because you took the refresher course?
   Yes _____ No _____
   What special problems or difficulties, if any, did you encounter in returning to practice? _____
   _____
   _____

(continued)

Exhibit 10.4 CONTINUED

Refresher Course Questionnaire

6. Work history since completing refresher course. Enter below in the appropriate columns the information requested about all the jobs you have held since completing the refresher course. Begin with your present job if you are working, or your last job if you are not working.

NAME AND ADDRESS OF AGENCY	POSITION	DATES EMPLOYED		NUMBER OF MONTHS DUR-ING WHICH YOU WORKED	AVERAGE HOURS WORKED PER MONTH
		FROM	TO		

7. Education

   School of Nursing from which you were graduated (Name and Location) _____

   Year Graduated _____ Additional education (Number of credits or degrees held): _____

   _____

   Have you had any additional education since completing the refresher course? Yes _____ No _____

   If "yes" Indicate: Number of credits completed _____

   Number of institutes attended _____

   Number of professional meetings attended _____

8. How far did you travel (one way) to take the course? _____ miles.

9. Would you encourage other inactive nurses to enroll in the refresher course? Yes _____ No _____

10. Have you encouraged other inactive nurses to return to nursing? Yes_____ No _____

11. What nursing literature do you use regularly? _____

    _____

    Are you reading more of the nursing literature since you took the course? Yes ___ No _____

12. Remarks:

The inactive nurse herself can provide helpful clues about the usefulness of course content. These may be sought by the instructor at the completion of the course, but throughout the entire course the instructor should adjust course content according to the enrollees' responses in discussions of their reaction to the experience and the extent to which the course is meeting each individual learner's own goals.

FUTURE DEVELOPMENTS

Societal changes have had and will continue to have an impact on the practice of nursing; several of these changes are directly related to the inactive nurse. The wider acceptance of part-time nurses and the increased opportunities for their employment are examples. This trend is very much related to the increasing numbers of employed married women in this country.

The graduate of a school of nursing today expects to combine marriage and a career; in the past, the female nurse was forced to choose between them. With the expectation that she will continue employment interspersed with short periods of inactivity, today's nurse will make an effort to keep herself professionally updated. Thus the need for refresher courses may eventually be replaced by a need for a continuous kind of professional education.

Continuing rapid technological advances will place increasing demands on nurses for keeping themselves informed on current professional practice. This will place greater demands on hospitals for more effective in-service education programs, but it will also require that educational institutions use more imaginative approaches and utilize newer media to get information to nurses during periods of inactivity. One approach using a state-wide telephone network (Fig. 10.2) is underway in Wisconsin. Others need to be developed.

The inactive nurse is a potential practitioner, but her return to practice may require several kinds of assistance. These include a well-planned refresher course, thoughtful job placement, a good orientation, and supportive supervision.

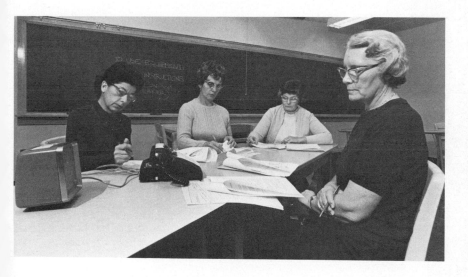

Figure 10-2 A statewide telephone network provides a way for inactive nurses in remote areas to keep informed of current developments in the profession. (*University of Wisconsin-Extension*)

An effective refresher course results from careful planning, effective teaching and selection of learning experiences, and extensive evaluation of results. The kind of courses currently being offered may not meet the requirements of the future and new approaches to helping inactive nurses keep current are now being explored.

REFERENCES

A Guide for the Establishment of Refresher Courses for Registered Nurses, American Nurses' Association, New York, n.d. (circa 1968).

"Back to Nursing," *Int. Nurs. Rev.*, **15**(2): 141-144, 1968.

Cleland, Virginia, Arnold Bellinger, Fredericka Shea, and Rosemary McLain: "Decisions to Reactivate Nursing Career," *Nurs. Res.*, **19**(5): 446-452, 1970.

Cooper, Signe S.: *Contemporary Nursing Practice: A Guide to the Returning Nurse*, McGraw-Hill Book Company, New York, 1970.

—————: "From Retired to Rehired," *J. Nurs. Adm.*, **1**(1): 24-28, 1971.

Davis, Marcella: "The Return Phenomenon," *Nurs. Forum*, **2**(2): 58-64, 1963.

Gessner, Barbara: "The Course That Refreshes," *Adult Lead.*, **15**(7): 229-230, 1967.

Hilkemeyer, Renilda: *Guidelines for Cancer Content in Refresher Courses for Registered Nurses*, American Cancer Society, New York, 1967.

Levine, Myra E.: *ReNewal for Nursing*, F. A. Davis Company, Philadelphia, 1971.

Marshall, Melody: "Refreshing the Refresher," *Amer. J. Nurs.*, **62**(11): 112-113, 1962.

McIntyre, Hattie Mildred: *Guidelines for Cardiovascular Disease Content in Refresher Courses for Registered Nurses*, American Heart Association, Committee on Nursing Education, New York, 1968.

Nurse Refresher Program Guide—from Start to Finish, Hospital Research and Education Trust of New Jersey, Princeton, New Jersey, 1967.

Reese, Dorothy: "How Many Caps Went on Again?" *Nurs. Outlook*, **10**(8): 517-519, 1962.

Refresher Programs for Inactive Professional Nurses: A Guide for Developing Courses of Study, U.S. Public Health Service Publication 1611, Washington, D.C., 1967.

Sparmacher, D. Ann and Maybel Wacker: "Their Caps Go On Again," *Nurs. Outlook*, **8**(1): 23-24, 1960.

Stryker, Ruth: *Return to Nursing*, 2d ed., W. B. Saunders Company, Philadelphia, 1971.

Tabler, Madeline: "Welcome Back to Nursing," *Nurs. Outlook*, **13**(9): 67-68, 1965.

11

In-service education

The cessation of learning is as real a threat to professional life as the cessation of pulse is to life itself. One of the ways by which the practicing nurse may continue learning is through educational opportunities which may be provided by his employing agency or institution. Traditionally called in-service education, this facet of continuing nursing education is of importance which cannot be overestimated. The intent of the following discussion is to provide an overview of selected factors which impinge upon any in-service endeavor and to consider some curriculum aspects in establishing an effective nursing in-service program.

Since the historical beginnings of in-service education were related in Chapter 2 they will not be repeated here. Yet one may be impressed with several implications from that discussion. For example, concerning the early years of preservice preparation for nursing, a question which might well be asked is "What are the real and actual differences between that preparation and what is now considered in-service education?" Another question is "Is in-service education as generally interpreted today still in process of evolution?" If change is accepted as a constant for life today, the response to the latter question must be "Yes."

A simple but commonly accepted definition of in-service education is that it is the educational opportunities provided by the employer for the employee to attain or improve his on-the-job efficiency, potential and capabilities. The translation from a simple definition to actual practice apparently is not so simple.

FACTORS AFFECTING NURSING IN-SERVICE PROGRAMS

The practice of nursing cannot be divorced from the health care industry. Neither can the educational efforts of a health profession be separated from the changes in the society which that profession seeks to serve. Thus the economic, social, medical, and technological sciences which affect that society will affect nursing in-service education.

Costs of Health Care

One of the pervasive problems in the United States for the last several decades has been the increasing costs of health care. A sharp upward swing in costs of all aspects of health care has been noted to include use of services, expenditures, personnel, facilities, insurance programs, and benefit payments.[1] Because health care costs are rising so rapidly and even though there are more health workers, including nurses, and more medical facilities than ever before in the history of the nation, there is a widespread and growing discontent with the obstacles to accessibility of professional health services.

While in-service education may be seen as a way to improve the efficiency of present services, some may view it as a source of another erosion on the debit side of the ledger which will necessitate adding to the costs of care. The question then becomes "Can we afford to have in-service education?" or "Can we afford not to have in-service education?"

Manpower

Although manpower in the health fields is increasing faster than the population, it is not keeping pace with the public demand. Between 1955 and 1965, the United States population rose by 17 percent; during the same period, the rise among practicing professional nurses was 44 percent. The rise among practical nurses and nursing assistants was 63 percent; the rise among physicians, 22 percent.[2] As the size of the population increases, the distribution of age groups changes, and a trend toward greater demands for health care is anticipated. By 1975, the health industry is predicted to become the nation's largest employer.[3]

The shortages in health manpower have been attributed to the rapid acceleration in building programs of hospitals and nursing homes without a corresponding rise in preparatory programs and a gross underestimation of demands from an affluent society.[4] As long ago as 1952 the prediction was that the expected supply of health personnel would not meet increased demands from new hospitals and expanding community health services.[5] Since then, the problems of health care have continued to receive intensive study and action on many fronts ranging from the federal legislative level to the local voluntary associations and agencies. If the decade of the seventies is truly the threshold for expansion of community health services, nursing in-service education will need to respond and correspond to those changes to try to maintain manpower needs.

Among the most acute shortages in nursing manpower is the supply of teachers prepared for teaching in nursing. Whether the teaching is to take place in an associate or baccalaureate or higher degree, hospital, or in-service program, nursing faculty with academic preparation in both clinical and functional areas are not in abundance. In fact, at least in one state, the faculty members for nursing in-service in general hospitals were often found to have their teaching responsibilities in addition to other full-time, primary service obligations.[6] Paradoxical as it may be, in in-service education where the greatest differences are found among the learners, and where the consequences of teaching are related to immediacy, the shortage of faculty manpower is most acute and likely to worsen as rapid changes in nursing practice occur.

Changes in Nursing Practice

As the practice of nursing broadens to include primary care or the maintenance of health in the well individual and extends to specialized areas such as coronary and intensive care units, knowledge of legal limits and safe practice cannot be neglected. Even though ideally, the teacher in the in-service program will have a command of some clinical expertise as well as of some adult education concepts, he need not be in addition a legal wizard. Rather, the teacher may guide learners to appropriate resources such as a local law librarian if there is one, or to textbooks such as *Law Every Nurse Should Know*[7] and *The Nurse's Guide to the Law.*[8] In addition the teacher may need to update himself, if that is appropriate, concerning his own legal responsibilities as an educator for nursing personnel in patient care and nursing practice.

That nursing personnel are busy people is seldom questioned. At least a partial reason for being busy may have been identified in a study which sought to discover the organizational patterns of nursing service existing in the nation's hospitals.[9] The Aydelotte report urged an inquiry into the organization of hospital services and identification of psychological, social, and economic forces which perpetuate current practices. For example, the provision by the nursing departments of continuity for other departments during evening and night hours and weekends results in a twofold function of nursing: nursing care to patients and continuity for other services.[10]

Another reason for being busy which may account for overt activities is that traditionally in nursing physical output was regarded as more efficient and desirable than intellectual productivity or purposeful interpersonal relationships with patients (see Fig. 11-1). Changes thought to be more responsive to needs in patient care are underway and are being studied. In one hospital the traditional nursing supervisory position was eliminated to provide clinical nurse experts who give and guide direct patient care.[11] More recently Esther Lucile Brown summarized and documented a number of changes which have occurred over time and which appear to constitute the establishment of some definite trends.[12] Brown cites the growth of formal in-service training as probably the

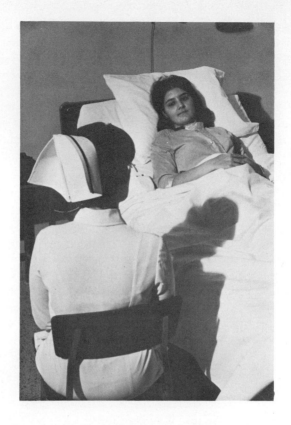

Figure 11-1 Purposeful nurse-patient interaction.
(Skot Weidemann, University of Wisconsin-Extension)

single most widespread development in nursing since World War II but cautions that since in-service faculty are in short supply, all possible resources for continuing education ought to be cultivated concurrently with in-service education.[13]

In England a group of six hospitals have combined under one director of nursing whose title is Chief Nursing Officer instead of the traditional Matron and whose responsibilities are for the nursing and midwifery services.[14] While certified nurse-midwives are not common across the United States, it seems likely that their numbers will increase along with other clinical nurse specialists and their expanding roles.

As mental health care becomes a part of all nursing practice, greater coordination among nurses from various settings is developing to provide continuity of care. Both inside and outside the hospital, nurses are being encouraged to communicate and coordinate their efforts from a highly specialized unit such as the intensive care unit to the general unit or between the hospital nurse and the public health nurse or the nurse from an extended care facility or a nursing home. When other common concerns of nurses, such as mental health care and continuity of care, are identified, coordination among practitioners undoubtedly will improve. One means of facilitating improved coordination is the establishment of standards for nursing practice.

Standards for Nursing Practice

Because the implications for meeting levels of expectation held for practice cannot be considered apart from in-service education, a brief review discussion will be included here. Standards for nursing practice have long been sought and are still in process of evolving.

In the early part of the 1950s Reiter and Kakosh conducted a study which attempted to establish valid, reliable, objective, and usable criteria for the appraisal of nursing care. Criteria were expected to be useful to hospital nurse administrators, nurse educators, and nurse practitioners because of the description of ongoing patient care. From the description the investigators hoped to derive indications of possible and desirable goals toward which the nursing profession might direct its attention.[15]

At mid-century, objective and observable criteria to assess nursing performance in patient care was a common concern. The American Nurses' Association (ANA) also embarked on a series of research projects on nursing functions. The research was subsidized by the nurses to evaluate progress in the provision of patient care. The comprehensive and final report of this series was published in 1958.[16] Other studies indicating a continued interest in this area have been reported by several investigators and are included in the list of references at the end of this chapter.

More recently, the ANA Committee on Nursing Service prepared *Standards for Organized Nursing Services in Hospitals, Public Health Agencies, Nursing Homes, Industries, and Clinics.* Then, the National League for Nursing produced *A Self-Evaluation Guide for Nursing Services in Hospitals and Related Institutions,* which reflected the standards enunciated by ANA. Each of the five Divisions of Practice in ANA, namely community health nursing, geriatric nursing, maternal and child health nursing, medical-surgical nursing, and psychiatric-mental health nursing are setting standards as a tool for use by the individual practitioner in self-evaluation of performance. Standards for nursing practice will assist in providing an operational definition of nursing and will undoubtedly prove to be useful to the in-service educator.

The Organization of the Nursing Department

Several of the recommendations in the report of the National Commission for the Study of Nursing and Nursing Education concern management and nursing administration. Included are specific references to planned orientation and in-service education courses.[17] Since it is obvious that organizational practices and policies as well as administrative support is important to the success of any venture in an agency or institution, an appraisal of the organization of the nursing department as it may affect in-service education may be useful. Rehm reports the reorganization at one large medical center to create and maintain a climate for learning and notes that changes were made in the organizational framework of the nursing department rather than in in-service programs.[18]

Whether the pattern of in-service education desired is to be the centralized, decentralized, or coordinated approach will be directly affected by organizational policies and practices. The centralized approach has its origin in the belief that the in-service curriculum ought to emanate from and be conducted by nursing personnel in the central administration of the agency. Conversely, the decentralized approach is based on a conviction that the in-service curriculum for all nursing personnel should be the responsibility, in large measure, of the practicing nurse with whom the personnel work. The coordinated approach is a compromise between the centralized and decentralized patterns in that, while the practicing nurse does indeed carry a large measure of responsibility for the in-service curriculum, the central administration nursing personnel of the agency is responsible for a broad program which is of import to all nursing personnel. In this way coordination is improved, duplication avoided, and unity of effort maintained. An added advantage of the coordinated approach is that, realistically, people will tend to lend support to an effort in which they personally participate or contribute; this approach involves both nursing administrators and practitioners in a complementary way.

APPROACHES TO IN-SERVICE EDUCATION

The pattern of in-service education developed within an agency may be a reflection of the organizational framework found there. For example, how likely is it that a centralized approach to in-service will be found in a traditional, authoritarian organization? Or, if the organization of the nursing service is more democratic than authoritarian, is it likely that either the decentralized or coordinated patterns of in-service will be found? A search for answers to such questions may be worthy of pursuit. While that investigation is outside the scope of this text, a consideration of each of the approaches may be of interest.

The Centralized Approach

Beyond the fact that nursing personnel in the central administration of the agency hold the major responsibility for in-service education, additional facts provide indications of a centralized approach. When none of the learners are consulted or participate in planning learning experiences and yet are expected to attend an in-service offering, a centralized approach is in practice. Likewise, when meetings are scheduled and solely planning and presented by administration to meet administrative needs, a centralized approach is obviously being used. For example, let us say that the nursing personnel have noted a recent rise in the number of diabetic patients in all areas served by the employing agency. The administrative staff have planned and scheduled an in-service meeting on interdepartmental communications. If the former group has any learning needs in relation to the care of the diabetic, those needs will not surface nor be met if the only in-service class is the meeting as planned.

A hazard of continued use of a centralized approach to in-service education is seen in reducing spontaneous, interested participation and enthusiasm of the learners. When learners are expected not to have much to contribute, they will inevitably live up to expectations. In-service that comes as a decree from on high may act like a vaccination. It may take but a little, yet it may provide immunity from further assault for a while. Probably the greatest single drawback to the centralized approach is that the in-service effort is assured only as long as central administration persists with it. When central administration is the fount and the fount runs dry, other wells do not come gushing forth without some preparation.

Some of the advantages to administration of a centralized approach are found when budget control and evaluation of programming are facilitated, when use of resources, people, places, and things are decided, and when committees are directed to work on specific problems identified by administration. Even though one or more committees may be appointed to gain representation from the employees or learners, the sheer existence of such groups does not guarantee an approach other than the centralized approach. The issue of which approach is being used is determined most easily by a consideration of the distribution in decision making for in-service education. If central administration makes most of the decisions that count, the outcome of the issue is not hard to determine. On the other hand, is it necessarily desirable that the learners make most of the decisions?

The Decentralized Approach

A decentralized approach may be familiar to nurses as unit in-service education or learning experiences related to the employee and the unit within an agency where the employee is placed. Although unit in-service may occur as a consequence of either the centralized or decentralized approach it is commonly equated with the decentralized approach. Decentralized in-service education is planned by and conducted for the employees of one or more units. The employees may be expected to keep administration informed of their activities and possibly consult with administration when help is wanted, but the employees are expected to develop and direct their own learning experiences. With a decentralized approach, control in planning for in-service is a responsibility of employees. If self-direction, initiative, and participation are qualities which are valued, they may be fostered by the decentralized approach. However, leadership, motivation, and creativity within the group will greatly influence the degree of group activity. Thus some of the disadvantages are readily seen.

According to the leadership provided within a unit, learning may flourish or fade. Then too, as a result of too little or too much enthusiasm, a group may tend to isolate itself from other groups on different schedules assigned to the same unit or to other units in the same agency. Team spirit is commendable but not if it disrupts the league. If problems are shared in common among units, concerted efforts to seek solutions are indicated. If solutions to problems are discovered, to share solutions is only logical.

Other disadvantages of a strictly decentralized approach vary from the apparent inefficiency of completely decentralized budgets or no budgets for in-service to the possible lack of availability of prepared faculty members for in-service education. Further, the units which are highly specialized are often the busiest units but also have the greatest needs for in-service among their personnel. Due possibly to changing technology or turnover of personnel which may occur in high stress areas, needs for in-service often remain unmet for nursing personnel assigned to such areas. Without knowledgeable guidance such as reported in an article by Coye, the situation will not improve with a decentralized approach alone.[19]

The advantages of a decentralized approach lie in that individuals who work on the same unit and confront problems in common share the responsibility for meeting in-service needs. The opportunities for face-to-face communications among the group of learners are more numerous than are afforded when one or two representatives of categories of nursing personnel appointed from a variety of units meet on call. Informal as well as formal planning, learning, and evaluation can take place with ease of communication in the same geographic unit or area. An expectation of a decentralized approach is that everyone will actively participate in the decision-making process to determine the direction of learning. In-service education which is relevant to the learner's concerns on-the-job is one result of such participation. Another result is the learning which may accrue to the individuals' benefit as they strive to identify with some precision the problem areas for learning on the unit. For example, if personnel tend to avoid or seem to dislike certain patients and know that their personal reactions to these patients may be voiced without censure or retribution, they may say such things as "He really bothers me" or "I can't stand him." Although the problem area may appear to be the patients concerned, the process to identify with some precision the problem areas for learning related to such situations may be useful—for instance: what do we know about the patient as a person,

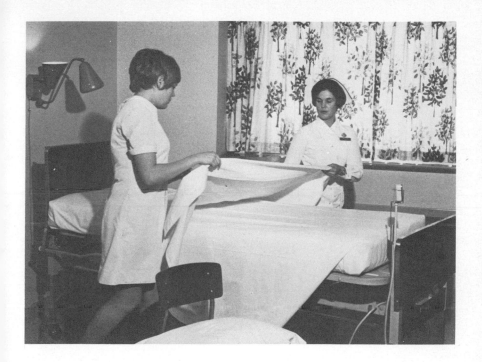

Figure 11-2 Nurse, as skillful role model, teaching a nursing assistant. *(Skot Weidemann, University of Wisconsin-Extension)*

what do we know about the patient's health condition or diagnosis, what do we
know about ourselves, and what else do we need to find out? Exposed to the
problem-solving approach over time, personnel may learn to integrate it with
their own reactions while focusing on a problem related to the employment
situation.

Immediacy is another advantage of the decentralized approach. Learning
on the unit from role models in the immediate work situation may be a subtle
but important form of in-service education for unit personnel. For those learners
who belong to the school of thought that says, "Don't tell me; show me," the
role models have impact (see Fig. 11-2). Even for learners who don't belong to
that school, the transition from cognition to behavior does not occur promptly
nor fully. Just as the essence of a problem may be difficult to identify, the value
of a role model's contribution to in-service education may be difficult to assess.
However, the potential for immediacy in learning in terms of time and place is
advantageous with a decentralized approach which includes all members on the
unit, some of whom are role models.

The inclusion of patients in the in-service education effort on the unit is facilitated with a decentralized approach. Hopefully the patient and the unit personnel know each other well enough to have developed some mutual trust and respect. Both are concerned with quality patient care. Patients, largely an untapped resource in in-service education, do have valuable and important contributions to make. Their thoughts, feelings, suggestions, responses and reactions require consideration in planning, conducting, and evaluating unit in-service and need to be systematically gained. In planning, for example, one question may be asked of every patient in the unit: "What do you think needs the least improvement and what needs the most improvement in this unit as far as help or services for patients are concerned?" The responses may indicate that personnel have a need to learn more about a particular aspect of services such as interpreting schedules if they cannot be altered or that a review of basic human or developmental needs of patients may be appropriate for personnel.

If teaching rounds are included as a way of conducting in-service, the patients may participate with minimal discomfort when the learners go to the patient rather than asking the patient to come to them. In evaluation the patients might be asked questions like "What is happening now that didn't happen before as far as schedules are concerned? Are people explaining things about the schedules better than they used to?" It may be that if patients are not accepting situations even with satisfactory modification of employee behavior from a previous situation, the problem-solving process must continue its circular course. In some instances the next step may be to help personnel work through their feelings of impatience with patients who reject the modified behavior or to identify more precisely the underlying problem of which schedules were merely a symptom.

A purely decentralized approach is theoretically possible but practically not probable for a prolonged effort. The pressures of getting the work done, time, willingness of people to become involved, turnover, and the lack of persisting leadership are factors which militate against it. However, once soundly established, it seems to have a better potential for continuation than does the centralized approach which comes to a standstill without direction from central administration.

The Coordinated Approach

When the strengths of the two approaches, centralized and decentralized, are adapted to formulate a third approach, the combination may prove useful. A total in-service education program which melds agency-wide and unit concerns in an appropriate way may increase efficiency and productivity of the effort. Rather than duplicating efforts or responsibilities, a coordinated approach provides for mutual cooperation and assistance to central administration and unit personnel in the agency. For the in-service education curriculum a central planning group, comprised of elected representatives from categories of person-nel and the in-service staff which is in a staff rather than line capacity, formulates short- and long-range goals and plans for the agency. An administra-tive advisory group comprised of chiefs in the agency serves as a consultative, informational resource to the planning group and as facilitator and expediter where and when cooperation is needed. For example, if the central planning group identifies a need to initiate an orientation curriculum in the agency, and if certain objectives for the course are best achieved through bringing employees from all units of the agency together, administrative support providing the opportunity and the expectation of attendance is helpful. If other course objectives are appropriate for unit in-service activities, administrative support for budget, time, and resources may be expected.

An orientation course provides a useful example for demonstrating the strengths of a coordinated approach. Every employee has some learning needs which he shares in common with other employees—such as agency personnel policies, fringe benefits, and the place of the agency in the community. Other learning needs are specific to his personal situation in terms of the unit to which he is assigned, its personnel, and service expectations. Thus a coordinated approach to meet learning needs is economical of not only the agency's but also the learner's time.

Because the in-service staff is readily available to consult on and foster unit in-service education, there is encouragement of communication, creativity, and experimentation with decentralized efforts. A coordinated approach may help fill in at least some of the gaps in educational leadership at the unit level. In addition a coordinated approach may make it possible for the learner to learn where the action is and where the patients are.

While the preceding discussion has touched on a number of selected factors which affect an in-service education endeavor in nursing, the following paragraphs will deal with thoughts on the process and development of the curriculum. Since much available literature on in-service education provides step-by-step guidelines such as those cited in the reference list at the end of this chapter, general approaches and considerations for the program will be included here.

CURRICULUM ASPECTS IN IN-SERVICE EDUCATION

Although the needs for continuing education and in-service education in nursing have long been realized, continuing education has been viewed by many nurses as taking place primarily within a formal academic setting.[20] In-service education tends to be regarded in a narrowly restrictive, vocational sense which is outside the concerns of either preservice or graduate education in nursing, and it is seen as the private concern of the employing agency. Yet Houle stated that the major education of the nurse should take place during the professional practice life of the individual, with a deliberate use of nursing experiences for learning purposes.[21] He suggested including a range of subjects outside of professional subjects to the end that the nurse may develop her intellectual powers to the fullest extent. If the inclusion of liberal studies is desirable and necessary in the preservice nursing curricula, any sound professional education may well emulate that concept.

In a number of agencies in-service education has consisted of two or three major components such as orientation, procedures and technical skills, and management or supervisory skills. As varied as the programs may be, the fact that nurses and nursing spearheaded in-service education in the health care industry is a historical feat. Even today an orientation program provided by the nursing department may be the only visible evidence of active in-service education in, for example, a small community hospital. Although there is a trend toward comprehensive in-service programs to include everyone employed within an agency, as found in industry, a point of pride may be that nursing was in the vanguard in the early planning and action on in-service.

Yet, with the modern advances in all areas of life and especially in the sciences, basic and applied, a review or modification of educational practices in line with research findings in education may be indicated. Do the traditional components of the in-service curriculum content need revision, in the light of shifting, changing conditions in the health field and in nursing? Will substitutions or additions be useful? Answers to such questions will depend upon the individual situation of each reader and the consideration given to the following curriculum aspects.

Who Is Involved

Although the faculty members and resource persons or experts who may be involved are important, individualized knowledge about the learner has the highest priority for relevant and effective program planning. Is the student ready to learn? What are his strengths and weaknesses? What are his experiences? What is his point of view? Has he learned to learn? What are his goals? Has he demonstrated motivation; in which situations? Of which groups is he a member? The more that is known about the learner, the better are the chances for tailoring learning experiences which are useful to him, individually or as a member of a group. If learning is seen as a change within the person and as a reorganization or restructuring of his framework of thought, he is the only one who can bring this about. The learner must be willing to engage himself. He is likely to be willing if his participation will result in a solution to or action on a problem which affects him or the people who concern him.

If a group is involved, knowledge about the individuals and the group are important. The group as a whole may initiate or develop goals, plans, or decisions which are far better than any one member of the group could have produced alone. For example, one of the problem areas in continuing education has been the difficulty in identifying learning needs. A tendency to base nursing in-service education solely upon the desires of the clientele is fairly commonly found. If a differentiation between wants and genuine needs for learning to improve services is made, a curriculum developed on the basis of stated interests alone may not suffice. Thus the group may be encouraged and guided to explore the relationships of stated interests of individuals to the improvement of the agency's or unit's services. All stated interests may not necessarily be legitimate content for inclusion in a curriculum. The reasons for the existence of an in-service program will be an influential factor.

Purposes and Objectives of In-Service Programs

From general education, much can be adapted to in-service education. Just as the purposes of an educational institution will provide direction for the development of specific objectives and curriculum content, so it is with a health-care agency. In education, the three commonly recognized sources of objectives are the content expert, society, and the learner. In nursing in-service education, another source requires recognition: the consumer of an agency's services. Together, the representatives from the four sources may profitably review and revise the purposes and objectives of the in-service program at regular intervals on an annual or biennial basis to keep them current, realistic, and appropriate for short- and long-term goals. Without a written statement of purposes and objectives, a program will lack a sufficient base from which to plan for a balanced approach to meet the learning needs. While a written statement is no guarantee for the quality, breadth, or depth of a program, it offers a documented stance which may be modified or improved for progress and evaluation.

The statement of purposes which includes the beliefs held for the roles of the agency, its personnel, and its clients, as well as the views held for the agency's service, education, and research functions in some detail, is likely to be more useful for program planning than a brief statement declaring generalized points. For example, to state that the agency recognizes that education of personnel is an important agency function is a general statement. Details, such as that the nurse has a right to expect that the educational program in the agency will assist him in increasing his personal and professional growth on-the-job, or the belief that every employee will benefit from continuing education offerings either within or outside the agency, add a clarifying dimension to the initial general statement. From an expansion of the detailed remarks, curriculum content areas may emerge. Traditionally the usual areas included in an in-service curriculum have been one or more of the following: orientation, skill training, management development, and continuing education. While these category areas for an in-service program may be practical and workable, so little is found in the nursing literature which deviates from the four areas that they may be suspect. Given the four traditional areas, do the purposes and objectives for a program derive from them rather than vice versa?

Just as there is lots of room at the top in nursing, there is lots of room for creativity in nursing in-service education and its curriculum development. Original and different approaches apart from the traditional may be valuable if soundly planned. Perhaps a problem-centered approach in considering agency, personnel, and client problems may be useful. Or a process approach, which uses the nursing process steps of assessment, planning, implementation and evaluation, then generalizes them to broader situations and different people, may be an appropriate way of proceeding from the statement of purposes and objectives. Should broad areas, such as communications, primary or distributive care, and secondary or episodic care, be considered as possible categoric areas for in-service education? Does skill training as applied to a specific program include manipulative or procedural skills only, or does it include managerial, interpersonal, and highly technical skills as well? While there is no right or wrong answer to any of the foregoing questions, thoughtful responses are needed to determine curriculum content and methods.

Curriculum Content and Methods

As an outgrowth of the carefully developed statement of purposes and objectives, concrete planning is in order. What are the content matters which will result in the knowledge, skills, attitudes and interests specified in the objectives? What are the methods, techniques, or devices which will need to be used for effective learning? Are content and methods related to the learner's life as he sees it? Will the opportunity to apply the new knowledge or practice a skill be present in the learner's real life situation? What are the resources for content expertise or for an efficient method for teaching-learning? Answers to these kinds of questions will help decide the concrete plans to be made.

In nursing, as in the biological sciences in general, content has been subject-centered. Perhaps subject-centeredness is unavoidable. One may question why a class on teaching the patient with diabetes is calmly accepted while one seldom hears of a class on teaching the patient with arthritis. Considering that arthritis is recognized to be the leading cause of chronic disability in the United States, what is the explanation? If content were focused on the process of teaching patients first, possibly in the centralized portion of the coordinated approach, then focused, at the unit or decentralized level, on individual patients for whom the learner cares, the content might have increased meaning for the learner.

Any discussion of content and methods needs to take into account the principles of learning, including a consideration of the sequence of learning experiences and the opportunities for the learner to relate to peers and faculty. With the variety of teaching-learning techniques available today the choices are greater than ever before. However the guidelines for selection remain the same.

Choices in selection of content, methods, and techniques are guided by an objective review of that which is known and by a search for additional ways and means in curriculum development. Then, from all the possibilities, selections are made which seem likely to aid in the achievement of learning objectives. Final choices are then made in terms of how the objectives may best be reached.

From the initial task of formulating the statement of purposes and objectives for an in-service education program, the placement of values on certain concepts of service and essential practices in health care was inescapable. Yet the importance of clearly identifying commonly held values is crucial for the establishment of a baseline for program evaluation. Ultimately, ongoing evaluation of a total program, in parts and as a whole, may well determine the future direction of that program.

Evaluation

Too often, the term *evaluation* has negative and terminal connotations. Personnel evaluations, for example, although intended to be constructive and helpful, are sometimes viewed negatively by both superior and subordinate. In relation to education, evaluation may be construed by some as a final examination which comes at the end of a course of study, with an implied threat of pass-fail. Both negative and terminal connotations do a disservice to the concept of evaluating the in-service education curriculum which is assisting the learner to attain, maintain, or improve his competencies. To be truly assistive, objective criteria mutually acceptable to both teacher and learner are set as benchmarks for the management of progress. Progress cannot be measured by one assessment at the end of a course. In a way, the facetious statement "How can I know where I'm going if I don't know where I've been?" has a basis in fact. Without knowledge of competency levels already held before a given set of learning experiences, difficulties will arise in measurement of progress, changes, or improvements in levels.

Occasionally, the banner of nursing in-service education is taken up with enthusiastic fervor by extremely action-oriented people who may mistakenly view the teaching-learning process as a panacea for all problems related to service. Planning for in-service may be regarded by these people as a minimally important facet, especially if the problem is an obvious one. Action toward a solution is likely to be taken with dedication and determination, but without a recognition that the behavior statement may indicate "We don't know where we're going but we're on our way." The consequences of such an approach for the evaluation of a total program are that the evaluation tools will not be any more systematic than the approach. Without design, organization, or system, any evaluation data collected are likely to provide a hodgepodge of information which may be interesting but of limited usefulness.

All who participate in designing the in-service curriculum are expected to contribute to the evaluation process within that curriculum. Evaluation is not solely the responsibility of the teacher. The identification of what is to be measured and the ways in which measurement will be achieved are determined by involving all who are concerned. Through the increased understanding and acceptance which may result from joint planning, the evaluation of learning is enhanced.

Although evaluation is concerned with the collection of objective data as measures of learning, the data are considered private and confidential information for educational purposes only. If in-service education is regarded as a truly educational endeavor, the learner ought to be assured of the confidentiality of his class performances. Line supervisors still retain the responsibility for counseling and appraising employee performance on the job, and test scores, attitudinal essays, or other educational data obtained in the class setting are not appropriate for any other uses. The focus on learning must remain clean and clear; the learning process should be guarded from infringement. Whether substantiation for a merit increase in salary or further basis for separating an individual from employment are sought, evaluation records of the learner's performance in the in-service curriculum are confidential.

Learning is a highly individualized and personal experience. Because of the individual differences among learners, the evaluation of a particular in-service curriculum may not be able to account for each and every learner's favorite mode of study. The learning approaches best suited to an individual may also vary according to the subject matter or the situation. Since self-directed learning is an important component of any continuing education, in-service or otherwise, the following chapter will consider that approach next.

Notes

1. Ronald Anderson and Odin W. Anderson, *A Decade of Health Services: Social Survey Trends in Use and Expenditure*, The University of Chicago Press, Chicago, 1967.

2. *Report of the National Advisory Commission on Health Manpower*, vol. I, U.S. Government Printing Office, Washington, D.C., 1967, p. 22.

3. Ibid.

4. "Crisis Ahead in Medical Care," *U.S. News and World Report*, February 26, 1968, p. 59.

5. *Building America's Health: A Report to the President by the President's Commission on the Health Needs of the Nation*, U.S. Government Printing Office, Washington, D.C., 1952, pp. 18-21.

6. May S. Hornback, "The Nature and Extent of Inservice Programs for Profession-al Nurses in General Hospitals in Wisconsin," Ph.D. dissertation, University of Wisconsin, Madison, 1969, p. 65.

7. Helen Creighton, *Law Every Nurse Should Know*, 2d ed., W. B. Saunders Company, Philadelphia, 1970.

8. Sidney H. Willig, *The Nurse's Guide to the Law*, McGraw-Hill Book Company, New York, 1970.

9. M. K. Aydelotte, *Survey of Hospital Nursing Services*, The National League for Nursing, New York, 1968, p. 1.

10. Ibid. pp. 2-3.

11. Louise Anderson, "The Clinical Nursing Expert," *Nurs. Outlook*, **14**(7): 62-64, 1966.

12. Esther Lucile Brown, "The Professional Role in Institutional Nursing," and "The Professional Role in Community Nursing," *Nursing Reconsidered: A Study of Change*, J. B. Lippincott Company, Philadelphia, 1970, Pts. 1-2.

13. Ibid., Pt. 1, pp. 76-78.

14. C. Biddulph, "The Changing Pattern of Nursing Administration in Hospitals," *Int. J. Nurs. Stud.*, **4**(2): 171-177, 1967.

15. Frances Reiter and Marguerite E. Kakosh, *Quality of Nursing Care: A Report of a Field Study to Establish Criteria 1950-1954*, Graduate School of Nursing, New York Medical College, New York, 1963, p. 122.

16. E. C. Hughes, H. M. Hughes, and Irwin Deutscher, *Twenty Thousand Nurses Tell Their Story*, J. B. Lippincott Company, Philadelphia, 1958.

17. National Commission for the Study of Nursing and Nursing Education, *An Abstract for Action*, McGraw-Hill Book Company, New York, 1970, pp. 123, 136.

18. Dorothy A. Rehm, "Design for the Staff Growth," *Amer. J. Nurs.*, **70**(9): 1930-1933, 1970.

19. Dorothy H. Coye, "What is Continuing Education in Nursing Service?" *Superv. Nurse*, **1**(6): 36-37, 39-40, 45, 48-50, 1970.

20. American Nurses' Association, *Avenues for Continued Learning*, The Association, New York, 1967.

21. Cyril O. Houle, "The Mind of the Nurse." A paper read before the annual meeting of the Chicago Council on Community Nursing, Chicago, March 12, 1969.

REFERENCES

ANA Committee on Nursing Service: *Standards for Organized Nursing Services in Hospitals, Public Health Agencies, Nursing Homes, Industries, and Clinics*, American Nurses Association, New York, 1965.

ANA Committee on Standards for Geriatric Nursing Practice: "Standards for Geriatric Nursing Practice," *Amer. J. Nurs.*, **70**(9): 1849-1897, 1970.

Anderson, Ronald, and Odin W. Anderson: *A Decade of Health Services: Social Survey Trends in Use and Expenditure*, The University of Chicago Press, Chicago, 1967.

Anderson, Louise: "The Clinical Nursing Expert," *Nurs. Outlook*, **14**(7): 62-64, 1966.

Aydelotte, M. K.: *Survey of Hospital Nursing Services*, The National League for Nursing, New York, 1968.

Biddulph, C.: "The Changing Pattern of Nursing Administration in Hospitals," *Int. J. Nurs. Stud.*, **4**(2): 171-177, 1967.

Brown, Esther Lucile: "The Professional Role in Institutional Nursing," and "The Professional Role in Community Nursing," *Nursing Reconsidered: A Study of Change*, J. B. Lippincott Company, Philadelphia, 1970, Pts. 1-2.

Building America's Health: A Report to the President by the President's Commission on the Health Needs of the Nation, U.S. Government Printing Office, Washington, D.C., 1952, pp. 18-21.

Coye, Dorothy H.: "What is Continuing Education in Nursing Service?" *Superv. Nurse.*, **1**(6): 36-37, 39-40, 45, 48-50, 1970.

Creighton, Helen: *Law Every Nurse Should Know*, 2d ed., W. B. Saunders Company, Philadelphia, 1970.

"Crisis Ahead in Medical Care," *U.S. News and World Report*, February 26, 1968, p. 59.

Dyer, E. D.: *Nurse Performance Description: Criteria, Predictors, and Correlates*, University of Utah Press, Salt Lake City, 1967.

"Establishing Standards for Nursing Practice," *Amer. J. Nurs.*, **67**(70): 1458-1463, 1969.

Germain, L.: "Nursing Service," *Hospitals*, **39**(7): 135-138, 1965.

Henry, N. B. (ed.): *Inservice Education for Teachers, Supervisors, and Administration: The Fifty-Sixth Yearbook of the National Society for the Study of Education*, Part 1, University of Chicago Press, Chicago, 1957.

Hornback, May S.: "The Nature and Extent of Inservice Programs for Professional Nurses in General Hospitals of Wisconsin," Ph.D. dissertation, University of Wisconsin, Madison, 1969.

Hospital Continuing Education Project: *Training and Continuing Education: A Handbook for Health Care Institutions*, Hospital Research and Educational Trust, Chicago, 1970.

Hughes, E. C., H. M. Hughes, and Irwin Deutscher, *Twenty Thousand Nurses Tell Their Story*, J. B. Lippincott Company, Philadelphia, 1958.

Jensen, A. C.: "Determining Critical Requirements of Nurses," *Nurs. Res.*, **9**(1): 8-11, 1960.

Johnston, Ruth V.: *Personnel Program Guide for Nursing Education and Nursing Service Agencies*, W. B. Saunders Company, Philadelphia, 1958.

Maxwell, R. Maureen: "The Preparation of Teachers of Nursing," *Nurs. Forum*, **7**(4): 365-374, 1968.

Mager, Robert F., and Peter Pipe: *Analyzing Performance Problems or "You Really Oughta Wanna,"* Fearon Publishers, Belmont, California, 1970.

Medearis, Naomi D., and Elda S. Popiel: "Guidelines for Organizing Inservice Education," *J. Nurs. Adm.*, **1**(4): 30-37, 1971.

Miller, Carol L.: "The Law and Nursing Education," *Educational Horizons*, **49**(2): 50-52, 1970-71.

Miller, M. A.: *Inservice Education for Hospital Nursing Personnel*, National League for Nursing, New York, 1958.

National Commission for the Study of Nursing and Nursing Education: *An Abstract for Action*, McGraw-Hill Book Company, New York, 1970.

National League for Nursing: *A Self Evaluation Guide for Nursing Services in Hospitals and Related Institutions*, National League for Nursing, New York, 1967.

Quint, J. C.: "Delineation of Qualitative Aspects of Nursing Care," *Nurs. Res.*, **11**(4): 204-206, 1962.

Rehm, Dorothy A.: "Design for Staff Growth," *Amer. J. Nurs.*, **70**(9): 1930-1933, 1970.

Reiter, Frances, and Marguerite E. Kakosh: *Quality of Nursing Care: A Report of a Field Study to Establish Criteria 1950-1954*, Graduate School of Nursing, New York Medical College, New York, 1963.

Report of the National Advisory Commission on Health Manpower, vol. 1, U.S. Government Printing Office, Washington, D.C., 1967.

Rudnick, Betty R., and Irma M. Bolte: "The Case for On-Going Inservice Education," *J. Nurs. Adm.*, **1**(2): 31-35, 1971.

Thomas, Lauraine: "Is Nursing Service Administration Prepared for the Professional Nurse?", *J. Nurs. Educ.*, **4**(1): 5-7, 1965.

Tate, B. L.: "Evaluation of Clinical Performance of the Staff Nurse," *Nurs. Res.*, **11**(1): 7-9, 1962.

Ujhely, G.: "Servants? No! Service Professionals? Yes!," *R.N.*, **27**(2): 55-60, 1964.

Willig, Sidney H.: *The Nurse's Guide to the Law*, McGraw-Hill Book Company, New York, 1970.

12

Self-directed learning

Ultimately each of us is responsible for his own continuing education. All education is really self-directed: what is learned and the extent of the learning that occurs depend upon the interest and the motivation of the learner, and the amount of effort expended.

This chapter explores the role of the continuing nurse educator in the encouragement of self-directed study. It assumes that the educator is himself a self-directed learner who serves as a role model to others. As emphasized elsewhere in this book, learning is a highly individual matter. Thus a significant role for the educator is to help each learner discover those approaches most useful to himself. To carry out this role effectively, the educator needs an awareness of many different approaches to learning.

Before the discussion of various approaches to self-directed learning, a consideration of personal planning may be useful. Available resources are of little value to the individual learner unless they can be used, and this implies planning for their use.

PLANNING FOR SELF-DEVELOPMENT

"Where do you plan to be five years from now?" was a question frequently asked of faculty members by a former dean of a midwestern school of nursing. She was helping them see the importance of setting goals and determining effective steps for reaching them.

Nurses are probably no different from other people; they may drift into various positions in their careers by accident rather than by careful planning. As a result nurses are frequently inadequately prepared for the positions they assume. This is particularly true when many opportunities are open to nurses, as in the period of time from the end of World War II to the present. The present state of affairs may be more serious in nursing than in other occupations because of the scarcity of prepared persons in leadership positions. Obviously such a situation is not good for society nor for the profession; neither is it good for the person, who may become thoroughly frustrated by his inadequate preparation for his job responsibilities.

Self-development relates to both one's personal and professional life, and in planning, both should be considered. Professional development includes all those activities that improve one's professional practice. Personal development includes activities contributing to personal growth and is so broad that it might range from learning to play the piano to reading good literature. Personal and professional development are closely interrelated, but the continuing learner plans for both.

Planning is the key to personal and professional development. It has been said that "we don't plan to fail—we just fail to plan." Placed in the proper perspective, planning may make the difference between success and failure in any venture.

Helping nurses plan for their own self-development is an important contribution of the continuing educator in nursing. Nurses know the value of planning for patient care so perhaps they need no convincing of the value of personal planning for themselves. Still it seems likely that most of us spend little time on this activity. Until recently basic nursing programs did not emphasize the need for continuing education to maintain professional competence, so nurses may not recognize the importance of learning as a lifelong pursuit.

Various planning formats, including some that are commercially available, may be useful, but as with nursing care plans, the format for the plan is not nearly as important as the planning itself. The format used by one nurse is given in Exhibit 12.1, but individuals may find that those which they design themselves are more useful to them.

The Planning Process

As with nursing care plans, the identification of both short-range and long-range goals is important to the individual. In this chapter a goal is defined as "an aim or end of action, a point to be reached."

Determining one's personal and professional goals is essential in a self-development plan. Each person must decide for himself what goals are important to him and establish their order of priority. Since learning is most efficient when goals are clear, adequate identification of meaningful goals is the first step in the planning process.

The determination of personal and professional goals need not be an elaborate process, but goals must be set with deliberate thought, and should be consistent with one's basic beliefs, personal philosophy, and life circumstances. They must be realistic for the person and attainable in a specific period of time. To assist the person in determining progress, they must be measurable to a substantial degree.

Exhibit 12.1 INDIVIDUAL PLAN FOR SELF-DEVELOPMENT

SELF-DEVELOPMENT PLAN

My plan for improvement in: *Oral Communication*

Starting date: *Oct. 20*

Things I can do:
1. Read on communication
2. Take a course
3. Make tape recordings
4. Increase my vocabulary
5. Seek opportunities to talk in public
6. Practice listening

What to do	How to do it	Target dates
1. Read "How to Talk with People", by Irving Lee	Borrow book from library	Finish by Nov. 1
2. Check University Center catalog for course offerings.	Note dates and plan work around them. Check registration date	October and November
3. Make tape recordings	Record for 3 min. and listen critically to playback	Oct. and Nov. — 3 times each week
4. Increase vocabulary	Scrabble; words in Readers' Digest. Work on crossword puzzles daily	Oct. and Nov. — weekly Oct. and Nov. — daily
5. Seek opportunities to talk in public	Offer services to Mental Health Ass'n. and church groups	First week in Nov.
6. Practice listening	Outline class, sermon or radio talk	Once a week in November

(Adapted from Norman C. Allhiser, "Self-Development for Supervisors and Managers." Used with permission).

Setting too many goals is a common error; inability to reach them causes frustration and a sense of failure. Setting realistic goals requires an understanding of one's ability. Many people do not make full use of their potential abilities; in contrast, others set their expectations beyond an attainable level.

Exhibit 12.2 STEPS IN SELF-DEVELOPMENT

1. Determine personal and professional goals.
2. Establish priorities for reaching goals.
3. Analyze use of available time.
4. Assess personal abilities and available resources.
5. Develop workable plan for self-improvement.
6. Evaluate progress at stated intervals.
7. Reassess goals and reorder priorities.

Setting meaningful goals and measuring the degree of attainment helps the person see progress. For example, when one identifies a goal as "to read more books," it is difficult to determine progress unless he understands what is meant by "more." A goal "to read 12 books each year" is easily measured; "to read six nursing books and six modern novels" is even more specific; identifying the books by name would be most useful of all.

It is usually best to establish time limitations for each goal. This limitation sets a definite time for evaluating one's goals and helps the person feel a sense of accomplishment with their achievement.

After goals have been determined, the next step in the planning process is an analysis of how one uses the time available to him. After this, assessing one's abilities and resources follows logically in planning, for any plan must be realistic and workable.

With the established goals in mind a workable plan of self-improvement can be outlined. The plan identifies possible approaches for reaching each goal, as illustrated in Exhibit 12.1. Each of us must feel a degree of success, so determining the progress that has been made is another important part of planning. As part of this self-evaluation, it is useful to reassess one's goals and priorities and adjust the plan accordingly.

Steps in the planning process are summarized in Exhibit 12.2. Planning can be as simple or as complex as the person wants to make it, but very elaborate planning is not necessary. Too extensive planning may be overwhelming and discouraging to the individual.

Time and Work Planning

"If I only had the time!" is a common complaint of most people. Because time is limited we need to learn how to use available time to best advantage. Using learning resources depends upon the availability of time. Although busy professionals often have time restrictions, careful planning will assure time for continued learning. It is a truism that we can find time for those things we want to do; when the person places a high priority on learning activities, he finds time for them.

An evaluation of how one's time is being used is the first step in planning time and work schedules. This requires keeping a detailed record of one's activities for a period of time—at least several days. Activities are recorded at 15-minute intervals, or other reasonable periods of time. After the recordings are completed a close examination of the detailed record will give a picture of the present use of time and provide clues to planning future use. This examination may suggest that the person needs to organize his work more effectively, search for time-savers, or delegate more activities.

Discovering ways of saving time on a specific job requires an assessment of the work itself. It is often appropriate to ask why we are doing a certain task; for example, needless records may be kept long after they have outlived their usefulness or when the information is available elsewhere. There may be simpler or more convenient ways of doing some nursing tasks. For some nurses time-savers may include learning to read faster, arranging one's work in a different order, or using the telephone more and dictating fewer letters.

Planning for one's off-work hours is also part of the self-development process. Again, records may reveal some surprises, such as the amount of time spent in making extra trips to the supermarket, or in coffee-klatches with the neighbors, or in viewing insipid television programs.

Effective advance planning of one's activities requires the identification of priorities. According to legend, industrialist Charles Schwabb paid a consultant $25,000 for the idea of listing job priorities in order of their importance. To attain goals it is necessary to determine priorities and to allocate time to those activities deemed most important.

Some planners suggest that the most difficult tasks of the day should be listed first in planning daily work; others believe that difficult tasks are best done during that time of the day in which the person works at his peak. Each person must discover which approach is most suitable for him, but setting tasks according to priority is a workable approach to effective planning.

The importance of planning for self-development cannot be overemphasized, for in our complex lives, there is often little time for individual and continuous study. Of course it is possible for a person to plan his time so completely (overprogram himself, in the parlance of the day) that his life lacks spontaneity. A good self-development plan is flexible and permits the person freedom to be spontaneous and creative, with time for relaxation and recreation.

Self-Appraisal

According to Socrates "The unexamined life is not worth living." Self-evaluation is discussed in more detail in the last chapter, but a few points are included here, for it is obvious that personal examination is an essential part of the self-development process.

Taking stock at intervals to identify activities important to oneself is a useful exercise. While we joke about making New Year's resolutions, the procedure of assessing oneself and setting new goals can be a meaningful experience, although more frequent self-evaluation may be desirable for many persons.

Individuals vary in their ability to recognize and assess their own capabilities and limitations. A greater emphasis placed on self-evaluation in basic nursing programs may encourage practicing nurses to continue the process throughout their professional careers.

Learning is enhanced by evidence of progress toward goals. Evidence of goal-attainment can be measured only when goals have been clearly defined. Self-appraisal has a useful purpose in helping nurses to measure progress and plan strategy for future development. Specific evidence of achievement helps the person feel a sense of accomplishment and motivates him to invest additional time, energy, and money in his continuing education. Thus continuing self-development depends upon continuing self-appraisal.

PERSONAL STUDY AND READING

The written word is the most frequently used and readily available source of information for most nurses. The reading of books and periodicals comprises the most obvious approach to self-directed study. Within the last decade the number of books designed for practicing nurses has increased substantially, as has the number of nursing periodicals. This rapid expansion requires that the nurse be selective in his personal reading.

Almost every nurse has access to the professional literature either through purchase or from lending libraries. The library as a resource and the various libraries available to nurses are discussed in the next chapter.

The dedicated learner subscribes to and reads those nursing periodicals of most significance to him. Such a nurse will discover additional sources of periodicals and other professional literature and probably will also seek out other types of reading. In all likelihood this nurse has his own nursing reference library, and makes appropriate additions at regular intervals.

The continuing learner in nursing does not restrict his reading to professional literature but reads broadly in many areas. This is a reflection of his interest in the world in which he lives, but it is also an appreciation of the value of good literature to one's understanding of people and their motivations, and thus contributes to his nursing skill. (It is interesting to note that the book section of the *American Journal of Nursing* thirty and more years ago listed many books other than those in nursing. Since nursing books were scarce, nurses were encouraged to read other types of literature, but perhaps there was also an early recognition of the value of reading broadly for the continued development of the practitioner.)

The amount of reading done by nurses is highly individual, but studies done at Ohio State University and elsewhere indicate that an awareness of the available literature motivates reading.[1] The implications for the continuing educator in nursing are obvious; informing nurses about available materials often encourages reading.

Implications for librarians are also obvious in these studies; colorful and clever displays and exhibits of recent books, pamphlets, and periodicals whet the reader's appetite. Through encouraging the use of various written materials, medical (and other) librarians are exceptional allies to the nurse who is in continuing education.

The increase in the number and the improvement of the quality of nursing publications is a boon to the nurse educator. These publications deserve a wider audience. Perhaps the nurse faculty member in continuing education as well as the teacher in the basic nursing program can make no greater contribution than encouraging the nurse to establish a pattern of reading the professional literature regularly.

AUTOINSTRUCTIONAL DEVICES

The rapid advancement of knowledge places demands on professional practitioners for keeping knowledge current. At the same time the number of employed, married nurses is increasing, so it seems imperative to identify flexible learning opportunities that can be adapted to the learner who cannot easily fit into the traditional educational system.

A number of teaching methods have been developed that are designed to present an instructional program without the presence of a teacher. Most of the approaches described here were not primarily designed for continuing education but can be adapted for this use. The independent approach to learning has a significant application to continuing education, particularly for the nurse who is a wife or mother bound to her home, or whose responsibilities are so great she cannot participate in other forms of continuing education, or who lives in a remote geographic area where educational opportunities are limited. The busy practitioner may not be able to participate in organized educational programs but can arrange a suitable time for independent learning.

Autoinstructional devices have many advantages. They promote learning by requiring active participation in the instructional process. The logical organization of materials also facilitates learning. If the tool is carefully designed, the learner is given immediate feedback, which serves to motivate him to further learning. It is an advantage to the learner to proceed at his own rate, which can be adjusted according to his ability and to the time convenient for him.

Autotutorial devices are often used to save instructional time, particularly when teaching demands frequent repetition. The preparation of these materials, however, is a very time-consuming process and requires considerable skill.

Programmed Instruction

Early developments in the use of programmed instruction were with teaching machines. The first of these, a testing device, was designed by Sidney Pressey in the early 1920s.[2] The current revival of interest came thirty years later, resulting from the work of B. F. Skinner in operant conditioning.

Programmed instruction is a student-centered method of instruction in which the information is presented in planned steps in carefully organized sequence, with the correct response immediately following each step. Programmed systems are based on the theory of reinforcement, discussed in Chapter 5.

Teaching machines of various kinds came into use early in the present development of programmed instruction, but today many programmed materials, including a substantial number in nursing, appear in printed form. To date only a limited number of programmed materials have been designed specifically for practicing nurses but more can be anticipated in the future. For readers not familiar with this educational approach to learning, some examples of programmed materials are included in the references at the end of the chapter.

As an independent approach to learning, programmed instruction has much application to continuing education. However the educator must be discriminating in selecting these materials, as with other learning aids. Criteria for judging quality programs include the accuracy and completeness of the content, the ease in following the directions, the appropriateness of the language for any specific learner, and the effectiveness of the items in teaching the concepts covered.

Computer-Assisted Instruction

Another application of the principles of programmed instruction is seen in computer-assisted instruction (CAI). Computers have the capability of storing information and feeding it back at a rapid rate; some can select previously prepared slides from an electronic slide sorter and draw letters and figures on an electronic blackboard.

In using computer-assisted instruction, the student sits at an electric typewriter console (Fig. 12-1), which is plugged into a central computer. After the student selects the desired program, the machine types out the first question and the student types in the response. If the response is correct, a second question is asked; if it is not correct, a question is posed to help the student arrive at the correct response. (As a last resort, the machine suggests, "See your teacher.")

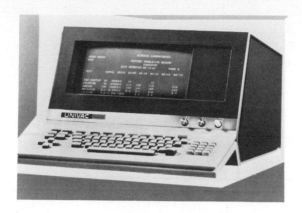

Figure 12-1 Console for computer-assisted instruction. *(Univac, Madison, Wis.)*

To date, materials in nursing designed for this type of instruction have been prepared for undergraduate students, such as that used in the PLATO simulated laboratory developed at the University of Illinois. The disadvantages of the system are the time and skill needed to prepare teaching materials for its program and the expense involved in its use. The system has obvious application to continuing education, since it can be used by learners in remote areas once materials have been designed. In the future more reliance will be placed on technology to assure the learner access to information.

Self-Study Units

Utilizing the principles of programmed instruction, a related self-study tool has been developed at the University of Wisconsin-Extension. Individual study units on selected nursing subjects have been prepared. Originally funded through the Wisconsin Regional Medical Program, the units were designed for inactive nurses, particularly for those who have limited means of keeping updated in the profession. The units were not seen as a replacement for a refresher course with clinical practice; rather, they are designed to help the nurse keep in touch with her profession during periods of inactivity. For the nurse planning a return to practice, selected units can serve as a preparation for a refresher course.

Each self-study unit is designed on a specific topic. Available units include nursing management of the patient with myocardial infarction, caring for the handicapped child, care of the comatose patient, and several others.

Each unit is designed in a way that its use requires the active involvement of the learner. The format includes a statement of objectives for the unit, a pretest to help the learner assess his knowledge of the subject, a study guide to direct his learning activities, various learning exercises with access to correct responses to permit testing progress, a poststudy examination, and a bibliography for continued study on the subject. Since participants may not have ready access to nursing information each packet includes appropriate reprints, pamphlets, and similar resource materials.

Although these self-study packets were designed for inactive nurses the tool has application for many areas of nursing. It can provide a review for the nurse who is changing to a different practice area. It can be adapted for group study, and serve as a basis for discussion for patient-centered inservice education. Additional study units designed for practicing nurses could also be developed.

Random Access Retrieval

For the busy practitioner, easy access to information becomes more critical as available knowledge expands. Several different approaches to retrieval of information are in use, and undoubtedly more will be developed in the future. Some very sophisticated systems of information retrieval have been established, primarily on college campuses. Retrieval systems appear to offer great promise for continuing education.

Television Retrieval Systems. The opportunity for playback of videotaped lectures has added a new dimension to education in a number of institutions. A television retrieval system permits students to see and hear content at convenient times or as often as necessary to understand it. In this system the student checks a directory for the number of the material he wants to view, dials the number on the telephone, and observes the playback.

Television retrieval systems require specially wired monitors. These are often placed in study carrels (Fig. 12-2), which may be located in designated study centers or in student dormitories.

The use of television retrieval has much potential for continuing education. The cost of the required equipment limits its use.

Telephone Retrieval Systems. Verbal information can be retrieved through the use of the telephone: Nursing Dial Access is one example of this type of retrieval. Modeled after a medical dial-access information system designed by Dr. Thomas Meyer at the University of Wisconsin in 1966, Nursing Dial Access was developed at the same institution through a grant from the Wisconsin Regional Medical Program.

Nursing Dial Access is a taped library consisting of short prerecorded audiotapes on selected nursing and related topics. The tapes range in length from three to nine minutes. By 1971 there were almost 100 tapes in the system.

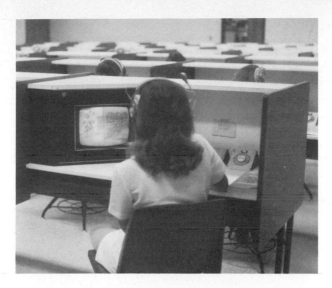

Figure 12-2 A television retrieval system permits the student to select a convenient time for study. (*South Dakota State University, Brookings*)

nurses also had access to the 500 tapes in the medical library. Additional tapes are being developed.

A nurse anywhere in Wisconsin may place a call from any telephone, at no charge to him. Nurses from outside the state may use the system, for the cost of a long-distance telephone call. The tapes have been purchased by medical centers in a few other states.

Requests to listen to a particular topic comes into the University's communication center (Fig. 12-3); the service is available twenty-four hours a day. The nurse requests the tape by its number, which he has in a list previously mailed to him.

In the communications center the access telephone is connected to a Cousino tape recorder. Tapes are on self-winding cartridges which are placed on the machine by the person answering the call. The recording stops automatically at the end of the tape.

A telephone dial access system has many advantages, although it has some obvious limitations where visualization would enhance an explanation. It has potential for getting recent information to nurses more rapidly than previously possible. Furthermore, it has the capability of reaching almost every nurse in the state, since calls can be made from the nurse's personal telephone.

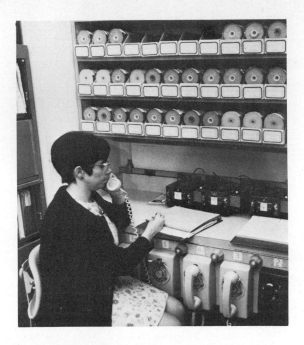

Figure 12-3 Requests for the use of dial access
tapes are handled at the communica-
tion center. (*Gary Schulz, University
of Wisconsin-Extension*)

The system has potential for providing information in many areas of
interest; general health information designed for the public is one of these.
Although the present arrangement is now operated manually, automating the
system is a possibility for the future.

Multimedia Learning Carrels

Only a brief mention will be made of the use of multimedia learning
carrels. More information is provided in Chapter 13, but much has been written
elsewhere on the subject, particularly as applied to the teaching of undergraduate students of nursing.

In many schools of nursing, students have access to multimedia learning
carrels (Fig. 12-4). They are designed for independent study using a variety of
media. Each individual unit may contain such items as a sound-slide projector
(or 35 mm slide projector with synchronized audiotapes), screen, tape recorder

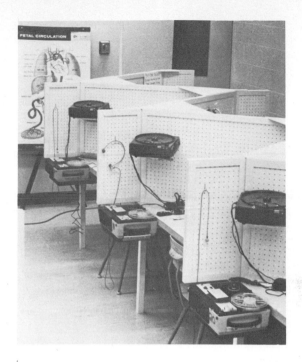

Figure 12-4   Multimedia learning carrels located in
a study center. (*Delta College, University Center, Michigan*)

single concept film projector, television monitor, and so on. Specialized units
include microscopes and other types of equipment.

The application to continuing education is apparent, although to date only
a few institutions provide study carrels for practitioners. Some of the learning
materials now available may be useful as a review for some nurses, but there is a
dearth of subject matter designed specifically for practicing nurses.

CORRESPONDENCE INSTRUCTION

Many nurses have rather a limited view on the value of correspondence
instruction. For some this attitude may have been colored by that period of time
when correspondence schools of nursing flourished in certain parts of the
country. Sometimes promoted by unscrupulous operators, these schools prom-
ised gullible students a career in nursing upon the completion of a correspon-

dence course. This era is not quite over; even today it is not unusual to see advertisements for correspondence courses for nursing aides or attendant nurses.

Excluding nursing and some other commercial fly-by-night enterprises, correspondence instruction has had a long and respected history. Many institutions of higher learning offer both credit and noncredit courses by correspondence.

In contrast to other forms of independent learning, correspondence instruction does involve a teacher, and the communication with the teacher is through correspondence. Minimally, the teacher's activities may be limited to reading and grading the student's assignments, but each lesson requires the personal attention of the teacher and the effective correspondence instructor devotes considerable time to each student. For this reason correspondence students get much more individual attention than a student attending a large lecture class on a typical college campus. However, students enrolled in correspondence courses often miss the stimulation provided by classroom discussion.

New tools, such as records and tape recordings, have improved some courses (foreign languages) or permitted the development of others (music appreciation) offered by correspondence. A combination of workshops with correspondence instruction has also enhanced the effectiveness of certain types of courses. An example of the latter arrangement is a course in nursing unit administration sponsored jointly by the Canadian Nurses Association and the Canadian Hospital Association.

The combined workshop-correspondence course in nursing unit administration extends over a seven-month period of time, beginning with a five day intramural session and ending with a similar offering. In the interim every student receives a series of twelve assignments, each of which is completed and mailed in for evaluation. In an effort to provide for individual guidance and assistance, the same instructor grades each student's work.

In contrast to some other types of correspondence study which permit more self-pacing, lessons are mailed to students at two-week intervals. Each assignment relates to the nurse's work situation, and may vary from a problem to be solved, or questions to be answered, to a project to be reported.

The Canadian program was funded by the W. K. Kellogg Foundation for a four-year period; since 1964 it has been self-sustaining. Kathleen Ruane was the first director and was responsible for developing the original materials; Dorothy Nelson now directs the program.

Since the first class registered in September, 1961, 4,543 nurses have completed the nursing unit administration course.[3] This includes 580 in the French-speaking section of the course, which has been in operation since 1962. Enrollees are in head nurse or supervisory positions while studying the program.

To accommodate the participants the workshops are scheduled on a regional basis in various parts of Canada.

Correspondence instruction does not lend itself to courses which require laboratory experience, such as the physical sciences and most nursing courses. However, a few nonlaboratory courses in nursing are available. For example, the 1971-72 Correspondence Study Bulletin of the University of Utah lists two nursing courses: orientation to nursing, and interpersonal aspects of nursing.

Sixty-two universities in the United States offer courses by correspondence. Listings of available offerings may be found in the *Guide to Correspondence Study in Colleges and Universities*, published by the National University Extension Association.

As a means of education, correspondence instruction has provided learning opportunities for many who otherwise would not have them: the housewife living on a farm 100 miles from the nearest college; the homebound ill or handicapped person; the lonely G-I serving at an outpost in India during World War II, or in Korea or Vietnam in more recent times.

For many nurses correspondence courses have provided a means of securing a number of college credits, particularly in the liberal arts, toward a college degree. It may also be the only opportunity available to the nurse whose working hours conflict with the time day courses are offered, or whose home and family responsibilities preclude her attendance at college.

The nurse planning to enroll in a correspondence course needs an awareness of the self-discipline required for this educational endeavor; the pressures of having to attend class at an appointed time are not present. The educator who has himself completed a correspondence course will appreciate the importance of this difference and interpret the need for self-discipline to the person who plans to pursue education by this route.

Correspondence instruction is a boon to those who do not have access to other kinds of continuing education, so it is useful for the nurse educator to be familiar with the many opportunities available. As nursing advances and knowledge expands, nurses themselves may demand more of these educational opportunities.

Correspondence instruction—alone or combined with supplementary educational approaches—has potential for upgrading nursing practice in underdeveloped countries. A combination of correspondence study correlated with information televised by satellite is one such possibility. International cooperation on educational programs for nurses desperately seeking new knowledge is an exciting challenge in the immediate future. Correspondence study provides one way of meeting learning needs that cannot otherwise be met and is a means for broadening and enriching the lives of many persons.

OTHER APPROACHES TO INDEPENDENT STUDY

Since individuals learn in different ways, the effectiveness of any independent approach to learning varies from one person to another. For many, variety also contributes to learning, so the development of new learning tools and new media appears to contribute to the learning process.

Several of the approaches mentioned in this section may be adapted to both independent and group learning but are included here since they are particularly useful for independent study. In these examples, learning materials specifically designed for nursing are very limited, but this does not preclude an eventual development of materials appropriate to the nurse learner. Also, the imaginative learner quickly recognizes nursing implications from many learning resources. One example: nurses wishing to improve their communication skills can apply content gained from a commercial listening course consisting of records and a workbook, even though the course is not specifically designed for nurses and has no specific nursing content.

Records and Audiotapes

Foreign languages were among the first subjects to be taught through the use of records, but with the advent of the tape recorder, opportunities for learning by listening have expanded. Learning by listening requires practice and some may find it difficult to concentrate on an oral presentation, particularly when no supportive visual materials are used with it.

A number of tapes designed for physicians for use in cassette recorders in automobiles have been commercially available for some time. A limited number of audiotapes appropriate for nurses have been released by the McGraw-Hill Book Company, the National League for Nursing, and other sources, and the availability of additional tapes can be anticipated.

Many nurses record their own taped libraries and share these tapes with colleagues. Easily portable tape recorders with very sensitive microphones have simplified the recording process. Reports, speeches from conventions and other meetings, and like materials can be recorded so that those unable to attend may hear the presentations. Often it is valuable to hear parts of a speech a second time to review what was said or to clarify points that were misunderstood or missed in the original speech.

Radio and Television

Like records and tape recorders, radio has the advantage of permitting the learner the opportunity of listening while doing tasks that do not require concentration. Thus the busy nurse housewife may find it convenient to listen while washing dishes or doing other household tasks. Some types of radio programs and recordings demand one's undivided attention, but this is not always true.

Two-way radio has been used in various parts of the country in providing educational offerings to nurses, but radio has the potential for greater use. As a teaching device it may be more effective when combined with a telephone arrangement, thus providing two-way communication. Its use is also enhanced when combined with correspondence instruction.

To date the most extensive use of open television in continuing education in nursing was the *Return to Nursing* series, designed as an integral part of a refresher course for inactive nurses. Produced under the direction of Marjorie Keenan by the Russell Sage College of Nursing the series was useful not only for its content, but in recognizing the potential of the medium in reaching large numbers of nurses. Individual study guides were developed to augment the learning of the viewers.

Under the leadership of Marjorie Squaires, educational television has probably been used more extensively in continuing education in nursing at the University of California at Los Angeles than elsewhere. Though most of the videotapes developed here were used as a basis for group discussion, they can be adapted for an independent study tool.

Television has potential for further expansion in the area of independent study. Eventually it will be possible for individuals to borrow or purchase cassette videotapes for use with their personal television monitor.

Personal Investigation and Self-Discovery

Little recognition is given to the learning that can occur on the job, but it is obvious that many nurses learn a great deal through seeking answers to questions that arise in the care of patients. The nurse with the inquiring mind learns through asking questions and in discussion with colleagues. Physicians and others are usually eager to share knowledge, and the nurse has only to indicate an interest to get some of his questions answered, thus adding to his fund of knowledge.

The hectic pace of many nursing units may make learning difficult for the individual nurse, but such obstacles will not block the real learner. Ready access to information, such as a small library on each nursing station in the hospital or the agency, will contribute substantially to his pursuit of knowledge and may motivate others to seek answers to their questions. Imaginative in-service educators have developed mobile libraries or traveling information carts (see Fig. 13-2) or developed eye-catching bulletin boards designed to encourage nurses to read nursing books or other references.

Study Centers

As nurses and others perfect their independent learning skills, there will be more demand for individual study centers stocked with a variety of learning tools. Hospitals and other employing agencies, as well as educational institutions, will arrange suitable places for practicing nurses to continue to learn. These centers may include individual study carrels and will provide easy access to the great variety of learning materials available to the nurse.

Notes

1. Alan M. Rees, et al.: The Structure and Function of the Hospital Library, *Hospital Administration,* **15**(14): 53, 1970.

2. "Sidney Leavitt Pressney, An Autobiography," *Leaders in American Education,* The Seventieth Yearbook of the National Society for the Study of Education, Part II, The Society, Chicago, 1971, Chap. 7, p. 246.

3. Dorothy Nelson, personal correspondence, June 11, 1971.

REFERENCES

Adams, Shirley: "A Self Study Tool for Independent Learning in Nursing," *J. Contin. Educ. Nurs.,* **2**(3): 27-31, 1971.

Allhiser, Norman C.: *Self-Development for Supervisors and Managers,* University Extension, The University of Wisconsin, Madison, 1967.

American Journal of Nursing, Selected programmed units in nursing, various issues, 1965-1967.

Bernzweig, Eli P.: *Nurse's Liability for Malpractice; A Programmed Course,* McGraw-Hill Book Company, New York, 1969.

Bitzer, Maryann: "Clinical Nursing Instruction via the Plato Simulated Laboratory," *Nurs. Res.,* **15**(2): 144-150, 1966.

Cooper, Signe S.: "Keeping Up with Nursing," *Contemporary Nursing Practice: A Guide to the Returning Nurse,* McGraw-Hill Book Company, New York, pp. 315-326, 1971.

Craytor, Josephine K., and Margot Fass: *The Nurse and the Cancer Patient: A Programmed Textbook,* J. B. Lippincott Co., Philadelphia, 1970.

de Tornyay, Rheba: "Instructional Technology and Nursing Education," *J. Nurs. Educ.,* **9**(2): 3-8; 34-35, 1970.

Frank, Sister Charles Marie: "On Continuing Growth," *Amer. J. Nurs.,* **60**(10): 1488-1490, 1960.

Gardner, John W.: *Self-Renewal: The Individual and the Innovative Society,* Harper and Row, New York, 1964.

Gerald, R. W. (ed.): *Computers and Education,* McGraw-Hill Book Company, New York, 1967.

Gleason, Gerald T. (ed.): *The Theory and Nature of Independent Learning,* International Textbook Company, Scranton, Pennsylvania, 1967.

Goldfarb, Martin: "Evaluation of the Extension Course in Nursing Unit Administration," *Canad. Nurse,* **62**(5): 59-61, 1966.

Hendershot, Carl (ed.): *Programmed Learning: A Bibliography of Programs and Presentation Devices,* 4th ed., Dr. Carl Hendershot, Bay City, Michigan, 1967-1968.

Horn, Ethel M.: "The Independent Study Tour," *Canad. Nurse,* **66**(1): 32-33, 1970.

Krueger, Elizabeth A.: *The Hypodermic Injection: A Programed Unit,* Teachers College Press, Teachers College, Columbia University, New York, 1966.

Lysaught, Jerome (ed.): "Individualized Instruction in Medical Education," *Proceedings of the Third Rochester Conference on Self-Instruction in Medical Education*, The University of Rochester, Rochester, New York, 1968.

_____: "Instructional Systems in Medical Education," *Proceedings of the Fourth Rochester Conference on Self-Instruction in Medical Education*, The University of Rochester, Rochester, New York, 1970.

_____: "Programmed Instruction in Medical Education," *Proceedings of the First Rochester Conference on Programmed Instruction*, The University of Rochester, Rochester, New York, 1965.

Lysaught, Jerome, and H. Jason (eds.): "Self Instruction in Medical Education," *Proceedings of the Second Rochester Conference on Self-Instruction in Medical Education*, The Rochester Clearinghouse, Rochester, New York, 1967.

MacKenzie, Ossian, Edward L. Christensen, and Paul Rigby: *Correspondence Instruction in the United States*, McGraw-Hill Book Company, New York, 1968.

Moore, Mary Lou: "Correspondence Courses for Registered Nurses?" *Nurs. Outlook*, 14(8): 45-47, 1966.

Niles, Anne: "Call 'Nursing Dial Access'," *Amer. J. Nurs.*, 69(6): 1235-1236, 1969.

_____: *Definitive Dialing—Nursing Dial Access*, University Extension, The University of Wisconsin, Madison, Wis., 1970.

_____: "Nursing Dial Access—A Taped Library for Professional Nurses," *Nurs. Forum*, 8(3): 328-36, 1969.

National University Extension Association, *A Guide to Independent Study Through Correspondence Instruction, 1970-72*, The Association, Washington, D.C., n.d.

Nursing Advisory Service of the National League for Nursing and the National Tuberculosis and Respiratory Disease Association: *Nursing Care in Tuberculosis: A Programmed Course of Instruction*, The League, New York, 1970.

Ruane, Kathleen: "An Extension Course in Nursing Unit Administration," *Canad. Nurse*, 57(1): 54, 1961.

University of Utah, Division of Continuing Education: *Correspondence Study Bulletin, 1971-72*, 62: 18, May, 1971.

White, Lucien W.: "Books and Reading in a Television Age," *Adult Lead.*, 14(7): 221-222; 246-248, 1966.

13

Resources for continuing education

Resources are often categorized as "men, money, and machines." A continuing education program is dependent upon all these items and each must be carefully considered.

Funding has been discussed previously in Chapter 6, so will not be considered again. This is not to deny that money is an essential resource. Keeping alert to potential financial resources is a responsibility of any continuing education program administrator who must develop some skill in obtaining these resources. The effective administrator places a high priority on securing adequate financial support.

This chapter will consider those resources which are used by the educator in designing and conducting programs and which are particularly useful to the learner. Some attention will also be directed to those resources that the educator himself uses for his own continuing education. Obviously there is some overlap between the two.

The skilled administrator knows how to make the most of available resources. But before this is possible he must be fully aware of those resources both within the educational institution and community and what they contribute to the program.

The most obvious place to begin to search for resources is in the institution itself. As educational institutions become larger it is increasingly more difficult to be aware of all these resources, so the educator may need to develop a systematic plan for keeping current about available resources.

HUMAN RESOURCES

Of all the resources available to the nurse in continuing education none is more important than people. The human element in the continuing education enterprise gives it a delightful variety and helps sustain interest, makes it stimulating and challenging, and certainly provides rewards and satisfaction.

Ideas are the lifeblood of continuing education. Since every person with whom the educator works can offer suggestions and ideas, every program participant is truly a resource. Flexibility in course planning provides the opportunity for participants to assist in establishing objectives and to modify course content on the basis of learning needs. Contributions from participants include ways of improving courses, suggestions for potential faculty, or ideas for the content of future offerings. Each contributes substantially to the overall continuing education program.

The flexibility of faculty members in the conduct of the program is encouraged by respect for the knowledge that program participants bring with them and the value of their experience in giving reality to planning and content. Use of the contributions of participants recognizes their worth as a resource to the program.

Advisory Committees

In most continuing education programs contributions by potential participants or some representative persons are sought in establishing advisory committees. Many different advisory committees exist: the department of continuing education may have its own advisory committee; there may be a statewide advisory committee; regional advisory committees may cover several states; an advisory committee may be set up for one specific course offering.

The composition of an advisory committee depends upon its purpose and the scope of its activities. Often general educators and other nonnurses are included. Some representation from practicing nurses results in more meaningful and realistic approaches.

A successful advisory committee depends upon careful selection of members. In this selection consideration is given to the person with a broad knowledge and understanding of current developments in nursing, with ability to work effectively as a member of a group, willingness to contribute time and effort to the committee, and ability to direct his attention to the future.

Faculty as a Resource

The selection of faculty members for a department of continuing education is discussed in detail in Chapter 7. The director of the department recognizes that the greatest asset he has is the faculty members with whom he works, and that one of his major responsibilities is assisting them in their own continued self-development. This in turn increases their effectiveness as educators.

This section is concerned with the selection of teaching faculty who do not hold full-time appointments in a department of continuing education but who teach in the program occasionally or on a part-time basis. These faculty members are selected for their nursing or other expertise rather than for their teaching abilities.

Nursing practice experts may or may not be skillful teachers. A nursing practice expert may need substantial coaching in the preparation of his presentation, in organizing content, and in selecting suitable supportive materials. He may need considerable support and assistance in the presentation itself; sometimes a team-teaching approach is most effective in assuring the best use of the knowledge of the practitioner. Often his greatest contribution is in the clinical setting, where he may be more at ease and more effective with informal rather than formal types of instruction.

In contrast to rather rigid institutional requirements for regular teaching faculty, considerable latitude is permitted in the selection of ad hoc faculty. This is advantageous in a continuing education program for it permits the appointment, albeit temporarily, of faculty with exceptional nursing practice abilities who may lack specific academic qualifications.

By his understanding of the problems faced by the practitioner, the nursing practice expert makes a unique contribution to the continuing education program. Approaches that are too theoretical or academic often have a negative effect on adult students; they need suggestions that have been tried and found effective. Because of their painful familiarity with the concerns of the real world of nursing practice, practitioners often learn best when confronted by a teacher who understands this world and is acutely aware of the problems they face. Counsel and assurance from an expert nurse is an effective teaching approach.

Depending upon the content of a particular course, faculty members other than nurses may be selected for specific course offerings. In helping nurses to learn to work more effectively in groups, for example, it has usually been necessary to search for appropriate faculty members outside of nursing, such as educators who are specialists in group dynamics. Physicians, pharmacists, and social workers—to name a few professional colleagues—can make special contributions in clinical nursing courses.

Unless they previously have worked extensively with groups of nurses, these nonnursing faculty members will need an orientation to the learning needs of nurses. It may be difficult to interpret to a physician the need to focus on content with specific application to nursing care, rather than to present merely a diluted version of a lecture for his medical colleagues. Nurses occasionally have difficulty in making application of general content, such as principles of management, to clinical practice. Therefore, whenever outside resources are used, program design should permit time for enrollees to consider ways in which content may apply to their nursing practice.

Locating potential faculty for a specific activity may require considerable ingenuity. If many part-time or ad hoc faculty members are used it may be desirable to develop some type of listing of potential resources. This listing would include general information, such as the person's location, as well as specific information about his education, experience, and particular area of expertise.

Suggestions for potential part-time faculty may be secured from colleagues, program participants, or members of advisory committees. The reactions of faculty members to speakers at conventions and other meetings may be another indicator of potential faculty. Deans and directors of schools of nursing, or other employers, may suggest members of their staffs when this information is requested, but may not always give an unbiased opinion.

Scanning the nursing literature may be productive in determining which persons have knowledge in specific practice areas, but additional information about the person's teaching ability is also required. Limited data about some potential faculty may be found in *Who's Who of American Women, Who's Who in Education*, and like publications.

Staff Support

A responsible clerical staff is another ingredient of a successful continuing education program. The clerical staff of a continuing education department must feel comfortable in meeting people. For many persons the initial contact with the department, either by telephone or in person, is with the secretarial staff. This public relations role may be a new one for many clerical workers.

When faculty members recognize the importance of the public relations role, they assist the clerical staff in every possible way in the effective performance of their functions. Chief among these is providing the staff with the information they need to be helpful to callers and to give requested information.

Telephone responses are indicative of the helpfulness of the clerical staff. The response to a telephone call reflects a personal interest; prompt attention to these requests is an important aspect of good public relations. Although the clerical staff cannot know the answers to all questions callers may ask, the staff can be expected to know where to get assistance in seeking the desired information.

In addition to the usual office skills of typing, filing, and transcribing materials, it is helpful if the clerical staff has additional skills. A certain amount of decision making may be required if faculty members are out of the office much of the time. Imagination and creativity are assets in the preparation of supportive material. Ability to plan work in advance and to work well under pressure may be necessary to handle the disparities in work loads resulting from unevenness in program planning.

Effective team functioning within a department of continuing education rests upon mutual respect of faculty and clerical staff. The clerical staff supports the faculty in every possible way in carrying out its teaching role. The faculty shows visible appreciation for the many contributions made to the enterprise by the clerical staff.

SUPPORTIVE SERVICES

The continuing educator in nursing in the college or university setting usually has access to a wide variety of supportive services. Experts in adult education are located in the extension service or the continuing education division; these adult educators are particularly valuable to the nurse whose educational preparation in this area is limited. The staff of tax-supported extension services can also provide assistance to those outside the institution in which they are located. The continuing educator in nursing, in whatever setting he works, will usually find it helpful to learn what is available to him through the extension service.

For the nurse newly appointed to a position in continuing education, it is helpful to get acquainted with resource persons early for assistance in program planning not available elsewhere. In addition, the resource persons are often very familiar with other local resources.

The staff of the continuing education division can be particularly helpful in assisting the nurse educator in broad areas of adult education, such as determining learning needs, over-all program planning, and evaluation. They can also contribute substantially in helping new faculty gain a familiarity with the supportive services provided by the university itself. Ideally this is part of his orientation to his position.

Supportive services vary from one institution to another and range from such mundane, but necessary, activities as addressing envelopes and mailing brochures to highly sophisticated computer services. Institutions usually provide for duplicating and printing, library support, publicity and public information. Institutional assistance in applying for grants and other financial support is discussed in Chapter 6.

Institutions may also provide more specialized services; these include assistance in photography and the graphic arts and in the use of radio and television. A number of universities have extensive audiovisual libraries. Often the nursing collection in these libraries is limited, but the staff of the audiovisual education or multimedia department has knowledge of resources and will search for additional films and other audiovisual materials.

Editorial services may be another specialized service provided by the institution not only in preparing fliers and brochures but occasionally in developing teaching materials and manuscripts. The collection and analysis of data for various kinds of studies is simplified with the provision of consultant and computer services.

Facilities

Although education may be possible with the teacher on one end of a log and the student on another, the adult educator knows that inadequate or uncomfortable facilities can interfere with learning. Most of us have experienced rooms uncomfortably hot or cold, or too crowded, or so noisy that the speaker could not be heard. Ideal physical facilities will not save a poor program, but many excellent programs have been spoiled by inadequate or uncomfortable facilities.

Attending to housekeeping details of program planning is a poor use of nursing time, but these details are so basic to good programming that they require extensive arrangements to assure their being done. No detail is too small to be overlooked. Many of these activities can be delegated by the nurse educator, who assigns each detail of program planning to a responsible person.

Arrangements for appropriate conference space is an important supportive service. In addition to planning for classrooms of an optimum size with the required teaching equipment and space for illustrative displays or exhibits, this service also includes provision for coffee breaks, special banquets and other meals, and social hours. Recreational activities may be planned as part of the program, particularly for one of more than a week's duration.

Many universities have specially designed conference centers (Fig. 13-1); most of the necessary arrangements for facilities are then handled by the center staff. Arrangements are even simpler if the conference center includes housing facilities; otherwise, the availability of hotel or other suitable accommodations must be considered.

Conference center personnel handle the housekeeping details of assigning rooms for planned sessions, arranging space for displays and exhibits, securing necessary teaching equipment and keeping it in good working order, and similar activities. A projectionist may be part of the center staff to handle films, videotapes, and other audiovisual presentations.

If the nurse educator has no access to this type of conference center and if appropriate facilities are not available in his institution, he must seek them elsewhere. It is wise to use care in selecting an appropriate location for education activities. The location should be easily accessible to participants; if it is an unfamiliar one, maps mailed in advance will help enrollees to find it. Housing accommodations should be nearby for those conferees who must arrange to live away from home.

In assessing any facility, costs must be carefully considered. Meeting rooms in hotels or motels may be available without charge, provided the enrollees are

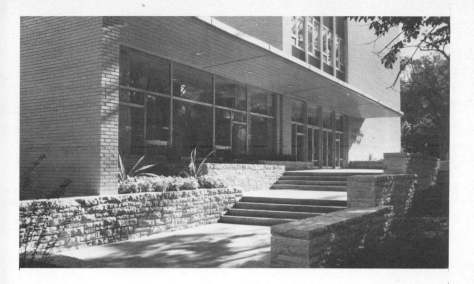

Figure 13-1   The conference center at the University of Wisconsin is one of many such facilities located in various parts of the country.

housed and take meals there. Another possibility is a meeting room in a public building, such as in a state-supported school or college or in a city library or museum. Increasingly, public buildings are constructed with the needs of adult learners in mind; meeting rooms may be heavily scheduled, so requests are required far in advance of the meeting date.

Banks and commercial concerns often have large meeting rooms that can be adapted for educational conferences; these are often available without charge. Many large hospitals usually have suitable meeting rooms, but sometimes the distractions from the call system or interruptions by staff participants leaving the session may preclude their use. Clinical courses require hospital or similar facilities.

The right type of facility contributes to the teaching program. Within the constraints of the educational institution in which he is employed, the educator must be selective in determining appropriate facilities for a particular offering.

LIBRARY RESOURCES

Books, periodicals, and other written materials remain the most easily accessible sources of information and continuing education tools for the largest number of nurses, in spite of modern technological advances and their application to education. The continuing educator in nursing must have an awareness of these resources and their location. This includes a familiarity not only with those resources available for his own personal use, but also with those accessible to the nurses with whom he works.

The quality and quantity of library publications vary considerably from one setting to another. Nurses in a large medical center frequently have access to a wide range of current periodicals and books; those in small hospitals, nursing homes, or public health agencies may have access to few, if any, publications. Nursing materials in many hospital libraries are often very scanty because nurses have not used available items or suggested the purchase of useful reference materials. An indication of interest as reflected in usage often makes the difference between a poor nursing library and a good one.

Sometimes nurses are not aware of library resources available to them. The nurse educator can assist in identifying these resources and in encouraging their use. In many instances the librarian welcomes suggestions from nurses for additions to existing collections, and the educator can encourage this kind of participation. In other instances the nurse educator may himself be in a position to suggest additions to a particular library.

Libraries in state tax-supported educational institutions may be one resource available to nurses throughout the state. Some medical libraries may be unable to meet requests for nursing materials, particularly as enrollments in schools of nursing continue to increase. Occasionally these libraries have small collections that are limited to out-state circulation; if they do not have such collections they may be encouraged to develop them with financial assistance. One example of such a collection was established in the medical library of the University of Wisconsin in Madison; books and related materials were purchased by the Wisconsin Heart Association for use by nurses with limited library access. Additions are made to this collection at regular intervals.

The nurse educator can often suggest other possible resources for nurses searching for appropriate materials. A local school of nursing is one example; although circulation of books may of necessity be limited to students, permission to use materials in the library will usually be granted to any nurse in the community.

The state traveling library is another example of a resource that may be overlooked by nurses. Nearly all states have a tax-supported reference library, but many do not have a nursing collection; this may be only because nurses have not requested materials from it. The nursing collection in the Wisconsin Loan and Reference Library was established in the 1930s, and remains an up-to-date collection. Originally nurses (and schools of nursing) could borrow only directly from the library; with improved library service today, the nurse now requests these materials through her local public library.

It is not without reason that the public library is sometimes called the people's university. With expansion of library holdings to resources other than books, the library has great potential for helping those with inquiring minds in their never-ending search for knowledge. Nurses may not recognize this potential of the public library.

Public libraries, particularly those in large cities, will often establish a nursing collection if nurses themselves initiate action and if the materials are used once they have been obtained. Sometimes a small nursing collection will be started in the public library by a donor, such as a district nurses' association or a local league for nursing. When the use of such a collection warrants expansion, the library budgets for additions to it. The nurse educator may suggest this approach to nurses who have difficulty in locating publications.

As discussed in the previous chapter, a small library in each hospital nursing unit may be the most useful of all libraries, since proximity to information is likely to assure its use. The in-service educator can encourage the development of small unit libraries and suggest those materials especially pertinent to each nursing station. In-service education departments sometimes establish their own traveling libraries (Fig. 13-2) with small collections of books and periodicals that rotate at specified intervals from one nursing unit to another.

The Nursing Literature

The impact of the knowledge explosion on nursing resulted in a proliferation of nursing books and periodicals. Of particular significance was the appearance in the late 1950s of books designed for practicing nurses. Prior to this time nearly all the nursing books were written for students. Practicing nurses were not book-buyers and consequently publishers did not seek authors of books suitable for the adult learner in nursing.

A number of new nursing periodicals have appeared in the last ten years, and as nursing becomes more specialized it is likely that additional ones will appear. Periodicals have a special place in the nurse's library since they often provide content of a different nature and information more current than that found in books.

The nurse educator has a responsibility to encourage practicing nurses to use the many written resources now available. Furthermore, he is often in a position to encourage nurses to share their ideas, suggestions for improving practice, or professional concerns through the written word. Improvement of the nursing literature requires capable and willing authors as well as discriminating and demanding readers.

Indexes. With the increase in the number of periodicals the retrieval of information becomes more complex. The busy nurse must be a discriminating reader, and this requires access to an appropriate index.

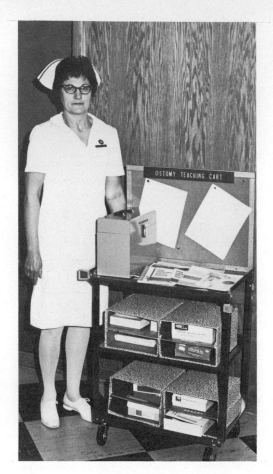

Figure 13-2   Traveling teaching carts are one way to make educational materials easily accessible to nurses. The materials are easily transported from one nursing unit to another. *(The Bismarck Hospital, Bismarck, North Dakota)*

The establishment of the *International Nursing Index* in 1966 was a particularly significant step for the nursing profession. This index is published at quarterly intervals with a final composite at the end of the year. For nurses without an easy access to library resources or for hospital libraries with extremely limited budgets, the *Index* might be the best investment that could be made.

Once the source of information is known, references can be located through other libraries. Many large libraries also provide a copying service so that single copies of articles can be secured at low cost.

The nurse educator needs a familiarity with other indexes in the field: *The Cumulative Index to Nursing Literature*, the *Nursing Studies Index*, the *Hospital Literature Index*, as well as the long-established *Index Medicus*. In addition it is often helpful to consult the *Education Index*, the *Social Sciences and Humanities Index*, and the familiar *Readers' Guide to Periodical Literature*. The *Nursing Studies Index*, a recently completed project under the direction of Virginia Henderson, is an annotated guide to reported studies, research, and historical materials. This index is in four volumes: Vol. I, 1900-1929; Vol. II, 1930-1939; Vol. III, 1950-1956; Vol. IV, 1957-1959.

The Medical Literature Analysis and Retrieval System (MEDLARS) of the National Library of Medicine is another important resource to the nursing educator and other nurses doing detailed study or research. The library serves as a national repository for biomedical literature, and the collection includes books, theses, journals, pamphlets, microfilms, and audiovisual materials. The automated bibliographic search service is usually requested through a medical library, as are requests for materials not locally available. These materials are often borrowed through regional medical libraries. A copy of the guide to MEDLARS services is available without charge from the National Library of Medicine (see reference at the end of this chapter).

Another important resource for the busy educator is the Educational Resources Information Center (ERIC). Funded by the U.S. Office of Education, ERIC is designed to facilitate and coordinate information storage and retrieval. The headquarters office is in Washington, D.C., with twenty clearinghouses located throughout the country. Each clearinghouse has responsibility for acquiring, indexing, and abstracting the literature in a given area of information pertaining to education. The ERIC Clearinghouse on Adult Education is located at Syracuse University.

Of special interest are two journals that print abstracts prepared by the ERIC system: *Research in Education* and *Current Index to Journals in Education*. Many documents indexed by the ERIC system not available from regular publishing sources may be purchased on inexpensive microfilm or in hard copy reproductions through the ERIC Document Reproduction Service (EDRS). Abstracts relating to research in nursing are published in *Nursing Research*.

The Librarian as a Resource

Many nurses may be unaware of the extent to which librarians can be supportive and helpful to them. The medical librarian makes an important, if indirect, contribution to patient care, so deserves recognition as a professional colleague.

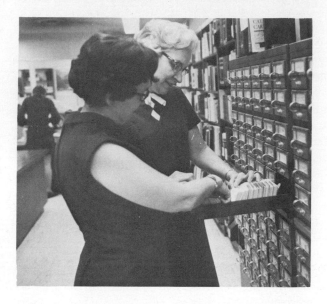

Figure 13-3 The assistance of the librarian in locating
unfamiliar resources contributes to the
continuing education program. (*Gary
Schulz, University of Wisconsin-Extension*)

A recognition of the librarian as a resource can save the nurse hours of
time in searching for necessary materials (Fig. 13-3). The librarian knows where
to locate references not easily accessible and how to use specialized libraries,
some of which the nurse may be totally unaware.

Some libraries provide extra services, such as the compilation of specialized bibliographies. In many situations, if the nurse makes his wishes known, the
librarian will be alert to items of particular interest to him and will direct his
attention to them.

A supportive librarian can make the job of the nurse in continuing
education much easier. In addition the educator must recognize the librarian as
an ally to all nurses and encourage nurses to take advantage of this resource.
Even in small communities an interested staff member of a public library can
contribute to the continuing education of the nurses in that geographic area.

AUDIOVISUAL RESOURCES

Machines were previously identified as a major resource; perhaps the
machines most useful to the nurse educator are those which contribute to the

teaching program. This includes a whole gamut of audiovisual equipment: 16 mm film projectors, 8 mm single concept film loop projectors, 2 x 2 slide projectors (with or without sound), overhead and opaque projectors, videotape players, and audiotape recorders. The use of selected materials in the teaching program is discussed in Chapter 8.

The effective teacher knows that he cannot always depend upon having the services of a projectionist, so he learns how to operate the equipment himself. This permits more flexibility in its use. Maintaining the equipment is usually the responsibility of the audiovisual education department; otherwise the educator should seek appropriate assistance to maintain equipment in good working order.

The need to be discriminating in the selection of materials has been emphasized with the development of increasing amounts of audiovisual materials. A number of resources can assist the educator in this selection process.

The most useful document for nurses is *The National Survey of Audiovisual Materials for Nursing*. A review of this compilation reveals that most of the nursing software developed to date is designed for undergraduate students. However, some of these materials can be adapted for practicing nurses, and more audiovisual aids for continuing education will be developed in the future.

Guides to Film Libraries

A review of film catalogs is a useful reference for the nurse educator. An extensive collection of these catalogs may often be found in the institution's library, but the teacher needs easy access to those he finds most useful for his program.

The catalog of audiovisuals and publications of the American Journal of Nursing Company is an important resource for any nurse educator. Many other film libraries also provide their listings upon request.

A number of state universities maintain film libraries where films can be rented for a modest fee. Film rentals may be limited to residents in the state, but this is not always the case.

State departments of health may also maintain film libraries; the use of these libraries is usually limited to state residents. The libraries are primarily geared to films for the public, but some films for professional audiences may be available.

The major voluntary health organizations, usually through their state affiliates, also maintain film libraries. Examples include the American Cancer Society, American Heart Association, National Association for Mental Health, and the National Tuberculosis and Respiratory Disease Association.

A large number of commercial concerns provide free films on loan. Many of these are high quality productions with advertisement kept at a minimum. As with many other films, preview before use is necessary to ascertain their value.

Exhibit 13.1   SAMPLE OF A FILM FILE CARD

<u>AUDIOVISUAL AIDS</u>

TITLE: *Mrs. Reynolds Needs a Nurse*

TYPE OF AID (FILM, VIDEOTAPE, ETC.): *Film; b/w, sound.*

LENGTH: *38 min.*

SOURCE: *Educational Services Division, A.J.N. Company*

SUMMARY: *Describes how a nursing care plan evolved for a "difficult" patient.*

USE: *Refresher course for inactive nurses; basic students.*

COMMENTS AND APPRAISAL: *Although the film is old (1964), the content is meaningful and stimulates good discussion.*

The nurse educator may find it useful to develop his own reference file on films and other audiovisual materials (see Exhibit 13.1). Information included in the reference file would be title of film, length, source, summary of content. An appraisal of each film and suggested use adds to the value of this reference file. Negative notations are also useful and can prevent the necessity for previewing materials a second time.

Free and Inexpensive Materials

In addition to having a familiarity with the usual library resources, the nurse educator needs some knowledge of the great number of pamphlets and similar materials available at little or no cost. These supplemental materials are often useful in teaching in a variety of ways: some contribute to the nurse's own knowledge, others are designed for the teaching of patients.

Many valuable materials have been developed by the nursing organizations, primarily the American Nurses' Association and the National League for Nursing. The voluntary health organizations, including those previously referred to, provide many useful materials in addition to films; these are usually requested through their state-affiliate associations.

The U.S. Government Printing Office has many useful documents for sale at low cost; lists of these publications are distributed twice a month to those requesting placement on the mailing list. Certain kinds of information may be secured from commercial concerns, such as insurance companies and pharmaceutical houses, usually without charge.

RESOURCES FOR THE CONTINUING LEARNER

Many resources are available for the continuing educator himself. An awareness of these resources and a plan for their use is necessary to his own continuing education. Among these resources are those found within his own institution.

Colleagues

We may not always appreciate the value of a colleague relationship to the learning process. For the nurse educator who works alone, it may be difficult to identify those persons who might be helpful; both nurses and nonnurses are possibilities. A nurse in a similar position may be ideal but not always available, and a respected and knowledgeable nurse in another position may be equally helpful.

Colleagues can serve as sounding boards for suggestions relating to continuing education for nursing. They help the individual in testing ideas, in exploring issues, and in sharing hopes, desires, and dreams. They provide support during periods of discouragement. Reassurance to the beginner in the field may be an especially important contribution. In a good colleague relationship, of course, support and testing ideas work both ways; it is the mutual acceptance and support of each other that contributes to an effective relationship.

In a department of continuing education, faculty are a resource to each other. In addition to the frequent spontaneous sharing that occurs constantly when faculty members are supportive of each other, it is also desirable to provide for more extensive opportunities for sharing concerns, exploring new approaches, and testing out ideas.

Professional Associations

Participation in the nursing organizations seems imperative to help the nurse educator keep fully aware of current developments in the profession. Participation in committee activities at all levels—local, state, and national—can be a learning experience for the educator and may contribute substantially to his general knowledge of nursing. Attending selected meetings and conventions also contributes to his continuing education.

Nurse educators disagree on the need for a separate organization devoted to continuing education in nursing. Alternative courses of action include an affiliation with the American Nurses' Association or the National League for Nursing, or the creation of a nursing section in one of the adult education associations. In 1972, the ANA Board of Directors approved the establishment of a Council on Continuing Education, designed to meet the need for continuing educators to share common concerns and to have a voice in decisions affecting continuing education in nursing.

An annual conference for nurses in continuing education is now offered, planned and sponsored by different educational institutions each year. In 1966 the faculty of the University of Wisconsin-Extension attempted to offer a conference for nurses in continuing education; only three persons indicated an interest in attending. Two years later, in conjunction with a national meeting for nurses in regional medical programs, the same university offered a one-day conference for nurse faculty members of educational institutions with continuing education programs. Thirty-four nurses attended that conference.

A burgeoning interest by nurses in continuing education was evident in 1969, when a national conference on continuing education was offered by the School of Nursing, Medical College of Virginia, Virginia Commonwealth University. Nearly one hundred nurses attended this conference held at Williamsburg. The following year the national conference was sponsored by Syracuse University and in 1971 the conference was held at the University of Wisconsin.

National conferences provide an opportunity for nurse educators with like interests to learn from each other. For the nurse new in continuing education, the University of Colorado has offered visitors' conferences. Formal sessions are presented and participants may also attend one of the regular continuing education offerings of the university.

In addition to participating in the nursing organizations, the continuing educator will want to know about and may wish to participate in some of the organizations that are more broadly concerned with adult education. Meeting experts in the field of adult education and sharing common concerns can be a learning experience for the nurse educator.

The Adult Education Association of the U.S.A. (AEA/USA) has been a leader among the organizations concerned with continuing education. Founded in 1951, the association now has state and local constituent units. Its stated purpose is:

> To further the acceptance of education as a process continuing through-out life; to afford opportunities to professional and nonprofessional adult educators to increase their competence; to receive and disseminate information about adult education; to promote a balanced development of educational services for adults; and to cooperate with educational agencies nationally and internationally.[1]

Adult Leadership, published monthly except July and August, is the official publication of AEA/USA, which also sponsors *Adult Education*, a research quarterly. The association also publishes a number of pamphlets and other materials useful to adult educators. Another of its significant publications is *The Handbook of Adult Education*, discussed on p. 235.

The nurse located in an extension division or other extension unit of a university will want to keep informed of the activities of the National University Extension Association (NUEA). Founded in 1915, the NUEA is an organization of educational institutions; its membership consists of more than 150 institutions. Its primary concern is to extend the resources of the university to meet the needs of an increasingly complex society. Members seek to develop, maintain, and advance sound educational practices in university extension, adult education, and public service.

Membership in the National Association for Public Continuing and Adult Education, (formerly the National Association for Public School Adult Education) consists of persons employed by public schools or state departments of education. A department of the National Education Association, the purpose of NAPCAE is to increase public understanding of public school adult education and to promote state and federal legislation in support of public school adult education. The organization provides a series of publications and holds an annual convention.

The Coalition of Adult Education Organizations (CAEO) was established in an effort to promote cooperation and coordination among organizations concerned with adult and continuing education. After much initial groundwork this organization was formally launched in January, 1970. Its purposes are to identify and focus on issues relating to continuing education, facilitate the exchange of information, act as a resource center for information, and promote support of adult education by the government, foundations, and other sources.

The American Society for Training and Development (ASTD) is primarily concerned with the practice of training and development in business and industry, but membership is open to other interested persons. It lists a number of nurses on its membership roster. *The Training and Development Journal* is its official publication. Local chapters meet at regular intervals.

Established in 1970, the American Society for Hospital Education and Training (ASHET) became the twelfth affiliate society of the American Hospital Association. Membership is comprised of educators and trainers of health care personnel and includes a large proportion of nurses. The development of state and local chapters is being encouraged.

In determining personal participation in organization activity, the continuing educator will need to be selective. Knowledge of the purpose of the organization and the scope of its functions and activities will assist in the selection process.

Exhibit 13.2   PERIODICALS ON ADULT AND
CONTINUING EDUCATION

ADULT EDUCATION. Research quarterly of the Adult Education
Association of the U.S.A., The Otis Building, 810 18th St., N.W.,
Washington, D.C. 20006.

ADULT LEADERSHIP. Published monthly (except July and August)
by the Adult Education Association of the U. S. A. (Address
above).

CONTINUING EDUCATION. Quarterly listing of short courses,
seminars, workshops in selected fields of interest. Indexed by
subject, location, and date. Data Bases, Division of Pennsylvania
Research Associates, Inc., 101 North 33rd St., Philadelphia,
Pennsylvania 19104.

CONTINUOUS LEARNING. Published bimonthly by the Canadian
Association for Adult Education, Corbett House, 21 Sultan
Street, Toronto 5, Ontario, Canada.

CONVERGENCE. International journal of adult education. P.O. Box
250, Station 5, Toronto 5, Ontario, Canada.

JOURNAL OF CONTINUING EDUCATION IN NURSING. Published
bimonthly by Charles B. Slack, Inc., 6900 Grove Road, Thorofare,
New Jersey 08086.

JOURNAL OF EXTENSION. Published quarterly by Extension
Journal, Inc. Edited by the National Agricultural Extension
Center for Advanced Study, University of Wisconsin, Madison,
Wisconsin, 53706.

TRAINING AND DEVELOPMENT JOURNAL. Official monthly
magazine of the American Society of Training and Development,
P. O. Box 5307, Madison, Wisconsin, 53705.

The Literature of Adult Education

The continuing nursing educator cannot function effectively without a
knowledge of the nursing literature. He will also find the literature in the field of
adult education an indispensable resource. In a constantly growing field it is
impossible to present an exhaustive listing of available resources, but some
suggestions are offered that may be useful, particularly to the nurse entering the
field.

To help gain perspective on the whole concept of continuing education, teachers may find reading some of the classics in adult education especially pertinent. A number of these documents are listed in the references at the end of Chapter 4.

Nurse educators will also want to be aware of the current literature in adult education. Several noteworthy periodicals were previously mentioned; a listing of periodicals pertaining to continuing education is given in Exhibit 13.2.

In a recently published book, *The Design of Education*, Cyril Houle has devoted over fifty pages to a review and commentary on the literature of adult education. This section of the book, entitled "Bibliographic Essay," surveys the field and is an excellent guide to both the neophyte and the experienced educator.

The Handbook of Adult Education, published by the Adult Education Association of the U.S.A., is a most useful reference. This handbook has appeared at intervals since 1934; the most recent edition is dated 1970. Proposed plans are to publish it every ten years. Much of the information found in issues prior to the last issue are also of general interest.

The Training and Development Handbook of the American Society of Training Directors offers many valuable suggestions to educators. *Training and Continuing Education: A Handbook for Health Care Institutions*, published by the Hospital Research and Education Trust, has more direct application to the hospital setting.

As its name implies, *Inservice Education for Hospital Nursing Personnel* proved to be a valuable reference for nurse in-service educators from the time it appeared in 1958. This classic handbook written by Mary Annice Miller for the National League for Nursing, was made possible by support from the W. K. Kellogg Foundation. Plans are now underway for updating this useful guide.

A familiarity with some of the research in adult education is useful to the nurse educator. Readers are referred to *An Overview of Adult Education Research*, by Edmund deS. Brunner, and to the quarterly publication *Adult Education*, discussed on p. 232. Research in continuing education in nursing is in its infancy but educators need an awareness of that which has been done.

Reports from early national and international conferences on continuing education in nursing are also useful documents. These are listed at the end of this chapter.

Notes

1. Robert M. Smith, et al. (eds.), *Handbook of Adult Education*, The Macmillan Company, New York, 1970, p. 530.

REFERENCES

American Journal of Nursing Company: Audiovisuals, Publications, Educational Services Division, AJN Company, New York, 1972.

_____: *The National Survey of Audiovisual Materials for Nursing*, Educational Services Division, AJN Company, New York, 1970.

Brunner, Edmund deS.: *An Overview of Adult Education Research*, Adult Education Association, Chicago, 1958.

Conklin, Colleen: *Guide to Nursing Resource Materials: Inservice Education, Heart, Cancer, and Stroke*, University of Michigan and Michigan Association of Regional Medical Programs, Ann Arbor, n.d.

Cooper, Signe S.: "The Nursing Literature," *J. Contin. Educ. Nurs.*, 1(3): 35-42, 1970.

Craig, Robert L. and Lester R. Bittel (eds.): *Training and Development Handbook*, McGraw-Hill Book Company, New York, 1967.

Curtis, Frieda Smith, et al.: *Continuing Education in Nursing*, Western Interstate Commission for Higher Education, Boulder, Colorado, 1969, pp. 57-64.

For Nurses Who Read, Department of Public Instruction, Division for Library Services, Madison, Wisconsin, 1970 (Mimeographed.)

Free and Inexpensive Materials for Use in Nursing Education, Department of Nursing, University Extension, University of Wisconsin, Madison, 1971.

Hospital Research and Educational Trust: *Training and Continuing Education: A Handbook for Health Care Institutions*, The Trust, Chicago, 1970.

Houle, Cyril O.: *The Design of Education*, Jossey-Bass Inc., Publishers, San Francisco, 1972.

Lembright, Katherine A.: "Continuing Education Program Within the American Heart Association," *J. Contin. Educ. Nurs.*, 1(2): 41-45, 1970.

Miller, Mary Annice: *Inservice Education for Hospital Nursing Personnel*, National League for Nursing, New York, 1958.

National Library of Medicine: *Guide to MEDLARS Services*, The Library, 8600 Rockville Pike, Bethesda, Maryland, 20014, 1969.

Smith, Robert M., George F. Aker, and J. R. Kidd, (eds.): *Handbook of Adult Education*, The Macmillan Company, New York, 1970.

Spector, Audrey F.: "The American Nurses' Association and Continuing Education," *J. Contin. Educ. Nurs.*, 2(2): 4-45, 1971.

Weldy, Alice: "Structuring for Continuing Education Within the Professional Association, *J. Contin. Educ. Nurs.*, 1(2): 36-40, 1970.

Conference Proceedings:

Cooper, Signe S. (ed.): "Critical Issues in Continuing Education in Nursing," National Conference on Continuing Education in Nursing, Oct. 18-21, 1971, University of Wisconsin-Extension, Madison, 1972.

McHenry, Ruth W. (ed.): "Ends and Means: The National Conference on Continuing Education in Nursing," *Notes and Essays on Education for Adults*, no. 69, Syracuse University Press, Syracuse, New York, 1971.

Proceedings Book of the National Conference on Continuing Education in Nursing, Health Sciences Division, Virginia Commonwealth University School of Nursing, Richmond, 1969.

Proceedings of the Conference on Continuing Nursing Education (First International Conference on continuing nursing education, McGill University, Montreal, Canada, June 24, 1969), Health Science Centre, School of Nursing, University of British Columbia, Vancouver, British Columbia.

14

Evaluating the effectiveness of the curriculum

To live today means living in an age of contradictions. On the one hand we hear that change is the sole constant of the modern age; on the other, we who are involved in any kind of education are continually exhorted to evaluate, to see if and what changes are occurring as if they might not occur. Previously, the teacher in continuing nursing education was identified as a change agent. This chapter will consider the implications for the change agent role as related to curriculum evaluation in continuing nursing education.

That the evaluation process is an integral component of curriculum development was repeatedly emphasized in other chapters. While a detailed discussion of the subject happens to be in the final chapter of this book, in no way do the authors relate the process to a terminal placement. Rather, the dilemma was like the age-old "Which came first, the chicken or the egg?" question. In a general way the first chapter which reviewed societal trends in health and nursing demonstrates an assessment of the society in which the curriculum develops. Thus that assessment may serve as an example of a part of the total educational evaluation process which encompasses all curriculum concerns.

Krug identified five societal concerns and needs related to the purposes and activities of education, namely to reduce the lag between technological and social progress; to promote individual self-actualization; to encourage democratic citizenship; to develop participation in the local community; and to establish a permanent peace in the world community.[1] Although Krug identified the needs more than a decade ago, they are still appropriate today. But what have they to do with evaluation in continuing nursing education?

No form of education can operate in isolation from the society it serves. The continuing nursing education curriculum and its evaluation need to take into account the goals of the large society as well as the goals which are immediate to the local community, sponsoring agency, clientele, and the particular educational effort.

While the concept of curriculum evaluation is in many respects abstract, complex, and perhaps difficult, the application and practice of the concept need not be intimidating. The concept is useful especially if the planning of the curriculum and its evaluation proceed in an orderly fashion. The purpose of curriculum evaluation is commonly accepted as involving measurements and judgments about changes in relation to particular objectives through teaching-learning. Thus the following section will focus on orderly ways of proceeding for a continuing nursing education curriculum evaluation.

THE PROCESS OF CURRICULUM EVALUATION

Evaluation as a process tends to follow a circular route when used as a feedback mechanism or guide to improve teaching-learning. Information about the degree, rate, or lack of changes may be obtained from evaluation findings. Also, unforeseen changes may be observed under some circumstances. However, the changes observed require some benchmarks such as antecedent knowledge, behavior, or skills for contrast to the present, or a scientifically derived speculation of prior levels of achievement related to present performance. The benchmarks are a means of measuring the progress and direction toward identified objectives. But who identifies the objectives and which ones are they?

IDENTIFYING OBJECTIVES FROM EDUCATIONAL PHILOSOPHY

The development of objectives ought to be a responsibility shared among all who are concerned with the curriculum. Objectives are too important to be left to one individual. The involvement of many points of view is necessary to develop an understandable and meaningful theoretical framework from which decisions about specific learning objectives can be made.

Although John Dewey defined philosophy as a general theory of education, the definition may be too vague, without the benefit of his further remarks, to be useful here.[2] But his definition serves to point out that the interplay between education and philosophy is vital and dynamic. While philosophy deals with theory and speculations, education deals with facts and practical applications. Each helps the other in a mutually reinforcing way. One without the other would suffer from the deprivation of extending ideas and feedback.

Because philosophers concern themselves with the study of the nature of knowledge and reality, precision in thought, and the basic values of society, they cannot be disregarded. A pluralistic society such as ours holds many differing and sometimes contradictory values. For example conflicting values such as "a good mother stays at home with her children" versus "a good nurse attends professional meetings," or "handmaiden" versus "creative professional" may affect where learning is to take place or what the objectives and content of the curriculum should include.

Whether knowledge is regarded as a tool or as an outcome of the educational process will differ with the philosophical stance. The difference may well determine whether subject matter or content is seen as adding to the quality of experience in the learning situation or as ends per se. Philosophy and education mesh at those points which involve very basic premises concerning man's existence in relation to knowledge and values, as well as premises concerning the general purposes of education which stem from those beliefs.

Because a discussion of other facets to consider in formulating an educational philosophy was included in Chapter 4, a repetition is not necessary here. An educational philosophy which addresses itself to particularly troublesome issues with clarity and precision will provide general guidance for curriculum development and evaluation. Furthermore, difficult decisions about objectives, content, and methods will become easier to make with theoretical bases clarified.

Identifying Objectives From A Psychology of Learning

A theory or psychology of learning which implies the systematic exploration of all aspects of learning grows out of an educational philosophy. Philosophical tenets are tested and the nature of the learning process is examined as regards their relationship to educational objectives and practices. A few of the concerns of interest to educational psychologists are touched on briefly here to provide examples of the relationship between theory and practices.

Individually, the teacher and the learner will have some kind of impact on the effectiveness of the learning process. For example, a teacher who relates well to people, has a sense of humor, enthusiasm, and good knowledge of subject matter, is skillful in conveying ideas, and can stimulate thought may have a beneficial effect on learning, while a teacher with opposite characteristics may not. Likewise, the learner whose readiness to learn, interests, and abilities lend themselves to the learning tasks at hand may benefit, whereas the learner with opposite characteristics may not.

Together, the teacher and the learner may affect each other and thus produce an effect on learning. The actions, interactions, and transactions of teacher and learner may well affect the motivations of either as well as encourage or discourage other facets of learning.

Since continuing nursing education is seldom carried on under a tutorial system where the instructor teaches one learner at a time, learning theory in relation to groups and group work is also appropriate as a resource in identifying objectives. The composition of a group, its sense of unity or disunity, and other characteristics which influence learning in a group have been studied by a number of investigators as cited by Thelen.[3] If learning theory based on research related to group instruction is reviewed as a part of curriculum development and evaluation, implications for teaching approaches and clientele may become evident.

Other important aspects of learning theory are associated with the total educational endeavor ranging from external forces such as community support which affect the curriculum to the detailed elements of physical settings and equipment used.[4] How content is learned, its relevance for the learner, the level or depth of understanding gained, and the effects of modes of content presentation, review, and practice are being systematically studied by educational psychologists. Researchers also include the study of human growth and development as an important area of concern. The impact that a psychology of learning has in identifying realistic or attainable objectives for a curriculum may be readily foreseen since the principles of learning are outgrowths of learning theory.

Defining and Refining Objectives

After the educational philosophy and the psychology of learning which are acceptable to the program planners have been determined, a comprehensive list of standards representing acceptable ideals or models of learning achievement is developed. The list of standards will reflect the theoretical bases in a practical way. Intensive thought, review, and attention are needed to develop a comprehensive list. There is no easy way. Omissions, contradictions, and additions require identification.

At some point either before or during the listing the standards may be categorized according to useful divisions, for instance: cognitive, affective, or psychomotor learning standards. These divisions may then be reviewed again to establish priorities and to determine which learning standards are essential and which are considered not quite as essential.

Starting with the most essential standard, criteria or specifications which will demonstrate progress toward or attainment of that standard need to be developed. These criteria are the set of expectancies or objectives which are to be developed through the curriculum and used for its evaluation. Minimally acceptable criteria as well as the criteria for ideal learning need to be explicit. Implicitly understood criteria which have not been explicitly stated compound difficulties in evaluation. Although the form and detail included in the criteria will vary according to the educational philosophy of the planning group, a consensus on what constitutes minimum requirements is necessary.

Simply that every expectancy held for a curriculum is impossible to identify or state precisely is not justification for foregoing the effort of defining and stating objectives. If the evaluation process is to be a systematic one, open to objective inquiry for the purpose of modifying and improving the continuing nursing education curriculum, a framework of clearly stated specifications is helpful. Clear statements are important because any education involves the communication process and communication at this level in planning will provide information, guidance, and support for the curriculum.

All who are concerned with the program need opportunities to consider, question, and validate the planning as it progresses rather than after its completion. The aspect of participatory planning is also viewed as a component of the shared accountability for the curriculum and its evaluation. The notion that one individual is solely responsible and accountable for the development and conduct of a curriculum is rejected. Not only the community and agency but also the teacher and the learners participate in defining objectives. Only in this way can a curriculum be developed in which the objectives are agreeable, understandable and acceptable to those concerned.

An occasional problem in nursing has been that some nurses have been more concerned with the form or format of team nursing, such as the Kardex form, than with the philosophy of its use. So it is with the definition of objectives. The form or detail of specifying objectives has sometimes overshadowed the concept of formulating objectives and considering their uses.

A cursory review of the literature of the kind cited in the references for this chapter reveals a range of opinions on the degree of specificity deemed desirable for written objectives. When there is no right or wrong answer, problems arise. For example, a generally stated objective such as "familiarity with dependable sources of information in nursing" may be no more right nor wrong than "given a list of ten titles from the nursing literature, the learner must be able to recall and name the author for each title." The former may permit somewhat greater flexibility in the teaching-learning process than the latter which implies that the course content must include at least ten titles from the nursing literature. Decisions on desired specificity of objectives will depend upon the planners, the situation, the subject matter or materials, and the analysis of standards.

Another way of defining some objectives may be by stating a task to be performed or a problem to be solved For example, "ability to associate urinary system physiology to selected nursing procedures" or "to be able to determine the amount of urinary retention by catheterization and measurement of residual urine" are objectives which imply performance. Again, in large measure, the flexibility envisioned within the curriculum will determine the detail possible to incorporate in the objectives. For instance, the first example permits greater flexibility for the teacher, the learner, and decisions concerning related content, materials, and methods to be used than does the second example. The procedure for catheterization to determine the amount of urinary retention and measurement of residual urine specifies particular subject matter and identified tasks, that is, catheterization, urinary retention, residual urine, and measurement. Whether one argues for the broadly stated objective or for a more specific and detailed objective, the criteria for the curriculum need to be defined, refined, and communicated not only for teaching-learning tasks but also for the curriculum evaluation.

Subobjectives may evolve as a result of the need to determine the most useful subject matter or the reasons why or how something needs to be learned. In the example given above, the second objective could be viewed as a subobjective for the first one. Objectives and subobjectives are the baselines for evaluative action.

Using Objectives For the Evaluation Process

Assuming that the objectives formulated are neither too broad to be useful nor too specific to inundate plans with minutiae, thoughtful decisions about what, when, and how evaluation will take place are in order. Should attainment of each and every one of the objectives be individually evaluated or is a representative sampling sufficient? What forms should the evaluation activities take? When and where should evaluation take place? The answers to such questions lie within the specifics of the objectives and the plans or blueprint for evaluation which are developed from the objectives.

In developing a blueprint for evaluation an analysis of the objectives is required to identify the inherent content or subject matter and the essential abilities desired as new learning. Shields discusses and illustrates a two-dimensional grid for the evaluation blueprint for a unit in geriatric nursing.[5] Although the analytic process to determine the content and ability or behavioral dimensions for a blueprint is a constant requirement, there are alternative ways of specifying plans for evaluation in a two-way table. For example, while Shields' blueprint includes particular identification of an objective in each cell of the grid, Payne's approach shows different ways of conceptualizing behavior and includes percentages in each cell to reflect the relative emphasis given each objective in relation to that total evaluation tool.[6]

Careful consideration of the content and behavioral aspects of the blueprint will provide cues to sequences for evaluation. If the entry level of attainment is determined before teaching is initiated, the objective which naturally follows the identified level logically provides a starting point. But, to know which objective naturally follows, the learner's expected behavior at the different levels of achievement toward an objective needs to be delineated. Inspection of the blueprint which contains these delineations will be helpful.

The next step in the evaluation process entails decisions on the settings and situations where the learner may best be enabled to demonstrate his learning. For example, returning to the previously cited objective concerning catheterization for residual urine, to test for that which is intended to be tested in nursing, the nurse caring for a patient requiring such treatment in the actual setting provides the most valid situation.

A simulated situation with a lifelike model such as a Mary Chase manikin in a mock patient care unit is valid but enjoys somewhat less relative validity than the real situation because a number of variables which may affect outcomes may be controlled. For example, if a subobjective specification concerns location and identification of the urinary meatus, the task is greatly simplified with a doll in contrast to a live woman. Verbal, that is, oral or written, descriptions of the placement of the meatus may also be clearly stated by the learner. However, describing is not the same as performing the procedure and so if performance is considered the most valid criterion for an objective, describing is less valid.

To enable the learner to demonstrate his learning, the evaluation settings and situations need to be as directly related as possible to the actual nursing situation where new learning is to be practiced. Factors which introduce artificial or distorting controls on learner performance need to be recognized and their presence reduced. The setting is weighed for its practicality and feasibility. Is it appropriate for the purposes of evaluation or is it so unique that another setting is indicated? Will the situation provide for an adequate sampling of the abilities learned to gain a consistent or reliable index of learning?

The forms that evaluation activities take today are limited only by the resources available to the instructional program and the imagination of the teachers and learners. Diagnostic, progress, and comprehensive examinations are possible using a variety of approaches. Teacher-made tests, role playing or dramatic performances, open or closed book tests, diaries, observations, filmed or videotaped situations calling for responses are just a few of the possible forms and approaches for evaluation. Yet, any or all of these are worthless without records of outcomes.

Records of Progress Towards Objectives

In continuing nursing education, a traditional concept of records which may be a carryover from earlier education in public and professional schooling is due for a change. Instead of a misplaced emphasis on grades or pass-fail, records are viewed as a reflection of progress towards curriculum objectives. Since the objectives are those which were developed and shared by the affected group in common, progress towards objectives is a mutual concern. Because the continuing learner in nursing is usually enrolled on a completely voluntary basis, his concern for learning is at least as urgent as the teacher's.

Thiede identifies three categories of records useful for evaluation and maintained respectively by the learner, an observer, or mechanical devices.[7] In the first category Thiede includes such tools as check lists, self inventories, and anecdotal records of behavior. A personally written plan for self-development and growth is another tool. In the second category he includes anecdotal records of observed behavior, interview records, and check lists of behavior. In the third category he includes audiotapes, films, videotapes, still photographs and graphic records of performance skills.

While categories of records are important, even more important is the realization of what the records themselves may represent. If a record is perceived differently by each individual who views it, the record may lack objectivity. For example, a nurse writes an anecdotal record of his own behavior, stating that a recently read professional journal article reported that a particular way of positioning a patient in a certain situation was a useful maneuver and that, on the basis of the article, the maneuver was employed by this nurse. One observer may view that action as prompt application of new knowledge while another observer may view it as a break with established procedure. When the goodness or badness of the record is objectively evaluated according to a mutually accepted objective, such as "is able to relate and apply nursing generalizations and conclusions to actual nursing situations," the seeming lack of objectivity decreases. Thus objectivity requires a framework for guidance. Objectivity also requires that other observers view a record in a common light with subjective appraisal at a minimum.

Records that are desirable represent a high degree of reliability as a part of the evaluation process. If a sampling of observations is limited according to time or span of variability so that other observers obtain different observations, the record may lack reliability. The consistency or agreement of different observers on observed behavior provides a measure of reliability in the records.

Although a record may be objective and reliable, the validity of a record is not ensured. For a valid record, the behavior intended to be represented must in fact be presented. For example, records of high performance on objective and reliable paper and pencil tests of knowledge on principles of asepsis and anatomy and physiology of the urinary system are not valid records of ability to perform catheterization. Because of varying degrees of validity which may be present in the evaluation effort, a striving for the greatest validity which may be present in the evaluation effort is desirable.

Records are of two kinds, personal and collective. Personal records of progress are maintained in utmost confidence between the teacher and learner. A collective record which summarizes outcomes in a unit, course, or curriculum and which does not identify the learners except as a collective group is used for class or course reporting purposes after it has been summarized.

Summarization of Evaluation

Without a summarization process, evaluation is incomplete. The myriad facts collected may well be meaningless unless they are systematically arranged, inspected, and analyzed. For example, the results of objective testing may be reviewed item by item to determine whether each item is in fact objective, valid, and reliable to serve the function that the total tool was intended to serve.

An item analysis may serve one or more of several different purposes:

To aid in the selection of items for improving a test.

To assess the objectivity, validity, and reliability of items or deficiencies of items.

To identify problem areas in learning for the collective group.

To consider areas of possible teaching deficits in instruction.

To assist the learner to identify personal problem areas in learning.

To identify expected outcomes which were not achieved.

To discover unanticipated outcomes which were not specified in the blueprint.

A variety of approaches to item analysis are readily available in current literature in the field of tests and measurement. Since the focus of this chapter is on the process of evaluation rather than techniques in measurement, further discussion is limited here. However, the notion of item analysis may have broader application than it has had in the past, when it was used primarily for paper and pencil objective test items. Adapting the approach to other evaluation records, such as anecdotal notes of behavior, may prove useful.

Descriptive summaries based on the prespecified criteria are another means of abstracting from the records an appraisal of progress. Writing a descriptive summary requires a careful review of the criteria and the records before items portraying important facets of performance are selected for inclusion in the narrative. At this point the criteria may need to be modified with additional specifications of levels between minimally acceptable and ideal performance. Does the level and the frequency of performance affect the viewing of outcomes? If so, those aspects are considered and delineated before the summary is written.

The summarization of evaluation involves collecting factual information, then categorizing, analyzing, and interpreting the evidence, and finally making judgmental decisions about the curriculum on the basis of all the previous activities. The judgmental decisions which are made will be in response to questions such as:

Are the curriculum objectives being attained and to what extent?

Which curriculum objectives are not being attained?

Do the objectives appear to be appropriate ones?

To what extent were the approaches viz. content, teaching-learning experiences effective?

To what extent is the learner being helped to meet his learning needs?

If the evaluation process was systematically well-planned and designed appropriately for the curriculum to be served, implemented, and followed through with care, the judgmental decisions are likely to be sound. They are apt to be not only objective, valid, and reliable but also useful to any nurse concerned with continuing nursing education. However, the evaluative decisions will be especially useful to the nurse educator because of the feedback gained in relation to the effectiveness of the nurse educator as a change agent via curriculum evaluation.

The process of curriculum evaluation as a shared effort is an important and practical means of promoting program improvements. When used, the concept serves as a demonstration of the educational accountability assumed by the community, sponsoring agency, instructional staff, and learners. Curriculum evaluation forms the basis and guide for modifying, revising, and improving the program. Yet not all continuing nursing education programs use the evaluation process consistently or as well as may be desired. The next section deals with some of the possible reasons for the foregoing observation.

SOME EVALUATION PROBLEMS IN CONTINUING NURSING EDUCATION

Even though some readers probably have the urge to say, "Don't tell me; let me tell you!" upon seeing the heading for this section, a review of the nature of selected problem areas may be helpful. From the administrative or instructional side, the demand for courses is often such that they should have started yesterday. From the learner's side, today is soon enough. Planning for evaluation is not really uppermost in everyone's mind. If that is the case, how can curriculum evaluation ever take place? The answer is, it cannot unless the long- and short-range planning for the curriculum includes the kinds of master or general plan described in the previous section as specifications, criteria, and objectives translated to a blueprint.

Without the framework for systematic evaluation of the curriculum, individual pieces of the curriculum, whether class, unit, course, or series of courses, can be appraised only in a haphazard way. Herein may lie an explanation for some of the difficulties in curriculum evaluation.

The Nurse Learner's Objectives

The nurse learner in continuing nursing education is usually a highly motivated enrollee who participates in the curriculum on a voluntary basis. (Mandatory continuing education will alter this situation.) Often the learner participates at some personal cost in terms of expense, time, and travel. Whether the reason for attendance is expanding professional interests or further preparation for nursing practice, the enrollee probably has a personal stake in being there. His objectives may be quite different from the objectives of others in the same group and may not completely coincide with the tentative teaching-learning objectives.

To promote involvement in the evaluative process as well as to provide a learning opportunity to understand better a systematic approach to the educational experience, discussion time allotted to development of mutually acceptable objectives is worthwhile. The learner may be confronting some immediate learning needs which for him are overriding needs. Unless these needs begin to be met the learner's readiness to learn other things may be unrealistic. To give an extreme example, if the nurse is concerned about effective means to keep a critically ill patient alive, a course on trends in nursing may appear to be totally unrelated. Yet if the nurse is encouraged to relate the care of the critically ill patient as an identified aspect of a trend in nursing like specialization and is guided to develop and extend his knowledge base in an area of interest, he may then be ready to attend to other facets of the course. With acknowledgment and acceptance of the learner's objectives, involvement in the evaluation process is enhanced.

Seldom are the objectives of nurse learners uniquely new in the sense of starting from a totally unknown base. His objectives usually build on previous knowledge and experience. The nurse adult educator and the learner together may wish to consider the cognitive, affective, and psychomotor aspects of mutually accepted objectives for meaningful evaluation. If the learner does not accept the instructional objectives he is not ready to learn. Opportunity to revise and modify the objectives together is crucial in allowing the learner and the nurse instructor to develop reasonable and responsible learning and evaluation within the framework for the curriculum.

Timing and Evaluation

Too often, evaluative activities are approached with the feeling that "It's got to be done." After one or another of the activities the unspoken thought may be "Well, that's done!" If evaluation is truly seen as appraising the value of the educational effort, it cannot be spasmodic or episodic; rather, it should be integral to the curriculum from its very conception.

Bloom differentiates between formative and summative evaluation.[8] He views formative evaluation as taking place along each stage of the educational experience, and summative evaluation as terminal. Bloom suggests that formative evaluation procedures be separated from the grading process and be presented primarily as aids for learning. Other effective uses for formative evaluation are for pacing student learning, promoting learner motivation, and probably most importantly, providing feedback to the learner and the instructor.

Depending on the length of continuing nursing education offerings, opportunities for formative evaluation may be limited. However, the concept is a sound one and merits serious consideration for planning to build it in where possible and practical.

Patient Care and Evaluation

If the ultimate goal of continuing nursing education is improved patient care, will a curriculum evaluation determine progress toward that goal? Again there are no easy answers. For a variety of reasons such as the particular objectives of teaching-learning, the practicality of evaluative activities needed, and ease or difficulty of follow-up in the clinical situation, outcomes of evaluation are likely to stop short of the ultimate goal. The assessment of patient welfare or improved patient care are difficult areas in which to develop reliable criteria. A more concerted effort is desirable than has been exercised to date to extend curriculum planning and its evaluation to the clinical area. Objective evidence of changes in a situation with many uncontrolled variables cannot be attributed only to the controlled variable of curriculum.

Rather than accepting that it cannot be done, the nurse instructor of continuing education can explore a virtually untapped field for research in associating evaluation of curriculum with evaluation of patient care. The body of nursing knowledge is expanding rapidly except in this particular area.

The problem is not unique to continuing nursing education. Its counterpart is likely to be found in the continuing professional education of any discipline. If preservice or graduate education had the answers, since they also are concerned with professional services, they could provide models. But models which tie evaluation of curriculum to evaluation of patient care are largely lacking or unidentified. Any steps taken in continuing nursing education to relate the two program aspects ought to be reported and shared.

The Nurse Learner and Self-Evaluation

Because the nurse learner is an adult learner who has his own goals and objectives, self-evaluation is a valid means to include in curriculum evaluation. Again the process may also be an educational experience for the nurse and useful to the learner in further self-direction of learning.

Somehow our society has tended to associate feelings of threat with the evaluative process. Whether the threatening feelings were engendered in an earlier stage of the educational process or in the employment situation, their existence is commonly recognized. Flunking out or failing to achieve a satisfactory performance level on a report cannot help but be viewed negatively by individuals. The problem in continuing nursing education may arise when self-evaluation implies penalty or reward rather than aid to progress in learning.

Preservice programs in nursing which encourage a self-evaluation process are apt to use a master form for particular courses which may not allow for very much freedom of response. As young adults the preservice students of nursing could be introduced to and helped to develop a method for self-evaluation to appraise their own progress toward their goals and objectives. Developing the ability to enhance internal aspects of evaluation through self-evaluation may be as important or more important than the imposition of external evaluative activities such as demonstrations of skills and tests for achieving both long- and short-range goals. Learners are no more ready to evaluate themselves on command than are instructional staff ready to evaluate a curriculum on command. Thus the nurse instructor in continuing nursing education may find that in many instances the learner may need to be taught the theory and practice of self-evaluation before the activity itself is included in the curriculum evaluation process.

While self-evaluation activities may not guarantee better learning, they may assist the learner to view his learning with increased objectivity or perhaps influence the level of his aspirations and affect his attitude toward learning. Self-evaluation as a process is another area that is ripe for research in continuing nursing education to explore its value in curriculum evaluation and improvement.

Evaluating Curriculum Components

A variety of offerings are likely to comprise a total continuing nursing education curriculum within a sponsoring agency. The offerings will vary in such aspects as objectives, content, clientele, place, instructional staff, methods of teaching-learning, duration, conduct, and evaluation that is practical or realistic.

Meaningful evaluation of learning from an offering of short duration is a problem for several reasons. If pre- and postlearning measures are sought, they are often difficult and expensive to obtain, perhaps impractical in terms of the time invested in the learning activity, and may not be warranted in view of the amount of change anticipated.

Refinement of objectives for offerings of short duration will help in the resolution of the problem. A limited number of precise and specific objectives may be more appropriate to use for evaluation than a global or ambitious set of objectives. If time is already short for the teaching-learning activities the time allotted to formative and summative evaluation will need careful budgeting.

Although the inclusion of evaluative activities is sometimes easier in a formally rather than informally conducted offering, inclusion is demanded. Mere reactions to a program reflect spontaneous feelings and may be only superficial indicators of response to the offering.

Evaluation cannot be left to chance. To ferret out the effectiveness of offerings in terms of learning, curriculum evaluation requires planning and implementation in each step of the way. As change agents in continuing nursing education, we will do well to heed Porter's caution that "If we fail to evaluate, while we may know exactly what we are doing, we will never know what we have done."[9]

Notes

1. Edward A. Krug, *Curriculum Planning*, rev. ed., Harper and Row, Publishers, New York, 1957, p. 2.

2. John Dewey, *Democracy and Education*, The Macmillan Company, New York, 1916, p. 383.

3. Herbert A. Thelen, "The Evaluation of Group Instruction," in Ralph W. Tyler (ed.), *Educational Evaluation: New Roles, New Means, The Sixty-eighth Yearbook of the National Society for the Study of Education*, The University of Chicago Press, Chicago, 1969, Pt. II, Chap. VII, pp. 115-155.

4. Herbert J. Klausmeier and William Goodwin, *Learning and Human Abilities Educational Psychology*, 2d ed., Harper and Row, Publishers, New York, 1966, p. 4.

5. Mary R. Shields, *The Use of Tests in Schools of Nursing The Construction and Use of Teacher-Made Tests*, 2d ed., National League for Nursing Test Construction Unit, pamphlet no. 5, New York, 1965, pp. 51-58.

6. David A. Payne, *The Specification and Measurement of Learning Outcomes*, Blaisdell Publishing Company, Waltham, Massachusetts, 1968, pp. 26-29.

7. Wilson Thiede, "Evaluation and Adult Education," in G. Jensen, A. A. Liveright, and W. Hallenbeck (eds.), *Adult Education Outlines of an Emerging Field of University Study*, Adult Education Association of the U.S.A., U.S.A., 1964, Chap. 15, p. 299.

8. Benjamin S. Bloom, "Some Theoretical Issues Relating to Educational Evaluation," *Educational Evaluation: New Roles, New Means, The Sixty-eighth Yearbook of National Society for the Study of Education*, The University of Chicago Press, Chicago, 1969, Pt. II, Chap. III, pp. 47-50.

9. John W. Porter, "Accountability in Education," *Accountability in Education*, Charles A. Jones Publishing Company, Worthington, Ohio, 1971, p. 46.

REFERENCES

Bigge, Morris L.: *Learning Theories for Teachers*, Harper and Row, Publishers, New York, 1964.

Blakey, Millard L., Irwin R. Jahns, and Wayne L. Schroeder: "The Case of the Self-Fulfilling Prophecy," *Adult Lead.*, **20**(6): 225-226, 1971.

Butler, J. Donald: *Four Philosophies and Their Practice in Education and Religion*, Harper and Brothers Publishers, New York, 1951.

Cantor, Nathaniel: *The Teaching-Learning Process*, The Dryden Press, New York, 1953.

Craig, Robert L., and Lester R. Bittel (eds.): *Training and Development Handbook*, sponsored by the American Society for Training and Development, McGraw-Hill Book Company, New York, 1967.

De Cecco, John P.: *The Psychology of Learning and Instruction: Educational Psychology*, Prentice-Hall, Inc., Englewood Cliffs, New Jersey, 1968.

Dewey, John: *Democracy and Education*, The Macmillan Company, New York, 1916.

The Evaluation of Teaching: A Report of the Second Pi Lambda Theta Catena, Pi Lambda Theta, Washington, D.C., 1967.

Furst, Edward J.: *Constructing Evaluation Instruments*, Longmans, Green and Company, New York, 1958.

Gronlund, Norman E.: *Stating Behavioral Objectives for Classroom Instruction*, The Macmillan Company, New York, 1970.

Hedges, William D.: *Testing and Evaluation for the Sciences in the Secondary School*, Wadsworth Publishing Company, Belmont, California, 1966.

Klausmeier, Herbert J., and William Goodwin: *Learning and Human Abilities Educational Psychology*, 2d ed., Harper and Row, Publishers, New York, 1966.

Krug, Edward A.: *Curriculum Planning*, rev. ed., Harper and Row, Publishers, New York, 1957.

Lessinger, Leon M., and Ralph W. Tyler (eds.): *Accountability in Education*, Charles A. Jones Publishing Company, Worthington, Ohio, 1971.

Mims, Fern H.: "The Need to Evaluate Group Therapy," *Nurs. Outlook*, 19(12): 776-778, 1971.

Monroe, Bruce, and Corinne Monroe: *Instructional Quality Control a Study Manual*, Objectives and Evaluations, Vol. 1, Instructional Systems Group, Inc., Long Beach, California, 1970.

Mortiz, Derry Ann, and Dorothy L. Sexton: "Evaluation: A Suggested Method for Appraising Quality," *J. Nurs. Educ.*, 9(1): 17-21; 24-25; 27; 29; 31-34, 1970.

Payne, David A.: *The Specification and Measurement of Learning Outcomes*, Blaisdell Publishing Company, Waltham, Massachusetts, 1968.

Popham, W. James, and Eva I. Baker: *Systematic Instruction*, Prentice-Hall, Inc., Englewood Cliffs, New Jersey, 1970.

Shields, Mary R.: *The Use of Tests in Schools of Nursing: The Construction and Use of Teacher-made Tests*, Pamphlet no. 5, 2d ed., National League for Nursing Test Construction Unit, New York, 1965.

Suchman, Edward A.: *Evaluative Research*, Russell Sage Foundation, New York, 1967.

Thiede, Wilson: "Evaluation and Adult Education," in G. Jensen, A. A. Liveright, and W. Hallenbeck (eds.), *Adult Education Outlines of an Emerging Field of University Study*, Adult Education Association of the U.S.A., U.S.A., 1964, chap. 15, pp. 291-305.

Topf, Margaret: "A Behavioral Checklist for Estimating the Development of Communication Skills," *J. Nurs. Educ.*, 8(4): 29-34, November 1969.

Tyler, Ralph W. (ed.): *Educational Evaluation: New Roles, New Means, The Sixty-eighth Yearbook of the National Society for the Study of Education*, Part II, The University of Chicago Press, Chicago, 1969.

Index

National League for Nursing, 27, 181, 210, 228, 229
National Library of Medicine, 225
National Survey of Audiovisual Materials in Nursing, The, 227
National Tuberculosis and Respiratory Disease Association, 227
National University Extension Association, 15, 209, 231
Needs, learning (*see* Learning needs)
Nelson, Dorothy, 208
New Haven Visiting Nurse Association, 22
New York League of Nursing Education, 24
News releases (*see* Publicity)
Neylan, Margaret, 33
Nightingale, Florence, quoted, 19
Nurse practitioner, pediatric, 12
(*See also* Extended role of nurses)
Nurses:
    as authors, 223
    clinical responsibility, 11
    clinical specialist, 11
    economic status, and fee payment, 94
    extended role of, 12
    inactive (*see* Inactive nurses)
    independent function of, 12
    life style, 8
    marital status, 7
    men, 8
    part-time, 169
    as professionals, 55
    shortages of, 178-179
Nurses' Associated Alumnae, 20
Nurses' association, district, 223
Nurses' Guide to the Law, The, 177
Nursing:
    audit, 136
    care plans, 136
    changing nature of, 10
    philosophy of, 55
    practice, 53
        changes in, 179-181
    team conferences, 150
Nursing Aide In-service Training Project, 27
Nursing Dial Access (*see* Random access retrieval; Telephone)
Nursing education:
    and authoritarianism, 51
    graduate courses, 151
    preparatory, 55
        and continuing education, 57
Nursing homes, 6
Nursing literature (*see* Literature)
Nursing Research, 225

Nursing Studies Index, 225
Nursing organizations (*see* American Nurses' Association; National League for Nursing; Professional Associations)
Nursing personnel, auxiliary, 11
    Red Cross volunteer, 26
    training of, 26-28

Objectives:
    for Conference on Health Maintenance Organizations, illus., 87
    for continuing education program, 87
    definition, 25
    of Department of Nursing, University of Wisconsin-Extension, illus., 86-87
    and evaluation, 240-241
    identifying, 140, 236-238
    of in-service programs, 189-190
    of learner, 245
    management by, 83
    secondary, 140
    for self-study units, 204
Off-campus teaching, 112, 113
Ohio State University, study on reading, 201
Older population (*see* Aging)
"Old Internationals," 31, 32
Operant conditioning, 77-78, 124
Organizations:
    health related, 106
    nursing, 2
        participation in, 110
    professional, 43-44
Organ transplants, 5, 165
Orientation programs, 8, 187
Overpopulation, 53
Overview of Adult Education Research, 233

Participants (*see* Enrollees)
Participation, and learning, 42, 51
Patient:
    advocate, role of the nurse, as, 55
    assessment, 132
    concern for, 55
    teaching, 6
Patient care, 246
    evaluation, 246
    planning, 196
Peace Corps, 55
Periodicals (*see* Literature)
Personal investigation, 211
Personal investigation, 213
Pfefferkorn, Blanche, 25
Pharmacist, in health teaching, 110
Philosophy, 47-59